CLINICAL NEUROIMAGING: CASES AND KEY POINTS

P9-ASL-866

David J. Anschel, MD
Assistant Professor of Neurology
State University of New York at Stony Brook
Associate Scientist
Brookhaven National Laboratory
Stony Brook, New York

Pantaleo Romanelli, MD
Responsabile, Neurochirurgia Funzionale, IRCCS Neuromed
Pozzilli, Italy
Scientific Director, Cyberknife Department
Iatropolis Clinic, Athens, Greece
Clinical Assistant Professor, Department of Neurology
New York State University at Stony Brook
Guest Scientist, Brookhaven National Laboratory
Upton, New York

Avi Mazumdar, MD
Interventional Neuroradiologist
Central DuPage Hospital
Chicago, Illinois

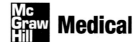

New York   Chicago   San Francisco   Lisbon   London   Madrid
Mexico City   Milan   New Delhi   San Juan   Seoul
Singapore   Sydney   Toronto

Clinical Neuroimaging: Cases and Key Points

Copyright ©2008 by The McGraw-Hill Companies, Inc. All rights reserved. Printed in the United States of America. Except as permitted under the United States Copyright Act of 1976, no part of this publication may be reproduced or distributed in any form or by any means, or stored in a data base or retrieval system, without the prior written permission of the publisher.

1 2 3 4 5 6 7 8 9 0   QPD/QPD   0 9 8 7

ISBN 978-0-07-147938-7
MHID 0-07-147938-4

This book was set in Times by International Typesetting and Composition.
The editors were Anne M. Sydor and Penelope Linskey.
The production supervisor was Sherri Souffrance.
Project management was provided by International Typesetting and Composition.
Quebecor Dubuque was printer and binder.

This book is printed on acid-free paper.

Notice

Medicine is an ever-changing science. As new research and clinical experience broaden our knowledge, changes in treatment and drug therapy are required. The authors and the publisher of this work have checked with sources believed to be reliable in their efforts to provide information that is complete and generally in accord with the standards accepted at the time of publication. However, in view of the possibility of human error or changes in medical sciences, neither the authors nor the publisher nor any other party who has been involved in the preparation or publication of this work warrants that the information contained herein is in every respect accurate or complete, and they disclaim all responsibility for any errors or omissions or for the results obtained from use of the information contained in this work. Readers are encouraged to confirm the information contained herein with other sources. For example and in particular, readers are advised to check the product information sheet included in the package of each drug they plan to administer to be certain that the information contained in this work is accurate and that changes have not been made in the recommended dose or in the contraindications for administration. This recommendation is of particular importance in connection with new or infrequently used drugs.

Cataloging-in-Publication Data for this title is on file with the Library of Congress.

International Edition 978-0-07-128723-4; MHID 0-07-128723-X
Copyright © 2008. Exclusive rights by The McGraw-Hill Companies, Inc., for manufacture and export. This book cannot be reexported from the country to which it is consigned by McGraw-Hill. The International Edition is not available in North America.

CONTENTS

PREFACE

While history and examination will always remain the foundation of neurological diagnosis, MRI and CT have now become the most important diagnostic tests used by neurologists and neurosurgeons. These tests are critical not only for confirming clinical diagnosis, but in many cases will give additional information absolutely essential to patient care. Modern clinical diagnosis and treatment of central nervous system disorders relies heavily upon neuroimaging. In some cases, the optimal management of clinical problems affecting patients with brain tumors, strokes, etc. depends on the ready detection of specific neuroimaging abnormalities. This trend will only continue to increase as more and more studies are based upon neuroimaging. Despite this fact, there is not an easy-to-understand book concerning this topic available for residents training in these specialties.

We found this situation rather frustrating during our own residencies and the idea for this book arose out of our desire to remedy the situation. Additionally, residents, especially during their early years, are the very first medical doctors to look at CTs or MRIs, frequently much sooner than the attending radiologist. Therefore, it is essential to recognize critical problems such as edematous brain tumors and bleeding, which require immediate action. This book has been designed for neurology, neurosurgery and radiology residents who need to have such a volume accessible. Residents will also find this book useful for exam preparation and understanding cases prior to rounding with attendings. We also hope this book will serve as an easy reference guide for those in these specialties already in practice. In addition, we hope that medical students, physicians in other specialties (for example, pathologists, family practioners, and internists, neurophysiologists, psychiatrists, and neuroscience researchers) will find this book useful due to the simplified and practical format as well as to the reference given to both normal and altered anatomy on neuroimaging studies. In addition to the most common clinical situations, we have chosen to include some of the rarer scenarios to emphasize the importance of remaining ever vigilant for these situations as well as to make the book more interesting.

David J. Anschel, MD
Pantaleo Romanelli, MD
Avi Mazumdar, MD

ACKNOWLEDGMENTS

The following individuals provided kind and generous assistance obtaining some of the images used in this book: Drs. Raphael Davis, Carl Hogerel, Arthur Rosiello, Mark Stephen, Wesley Carrion, Katie Vo, Robert Galler, and Ronald Budzik.

Part 1

INTRODUCTION

Chapter 1

BASICS OF MRI AND CT PHYSICS

Magnetic resonance imaging (MRI) creates images by exploiting the magnetic properties of protons in the body, using the application of magnetic fields and a radiofrequency pulse.

Certain elements, with an odd number of protons or neutrons, will have magnetic properties when placed in a magnetic field. Because protons are found in large numbers in the human body (primarily within water), they are the most useful for imaging.

Protons are generally aligned in random directions (see Fig. 1-1). MRI scanners have a standing magnetic field oriented along the longitudinal direction of the bore of the magnet (B_o). When placed in this magnetic field, protons will precess (spin) in a parallel (low energy/α-spin state) or antiparallel orientation (high energy/β-spin state) (see Fig. 1-2).

The frequency of precession is known as the *larmor frequency* and depends on the strength of the local magnetic field. The main magnetic field (by convention noted as the Z-direction) is applied to align magnetic spins along the long axis of the body.

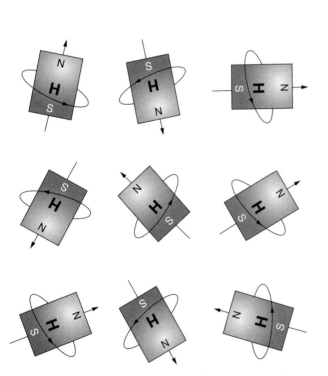

FIG. 1-1 In their resting state, protons have a random orientation with a zero net magnetization. Each proton can be thought of as a magnet with a north (N) and south (S) pole.

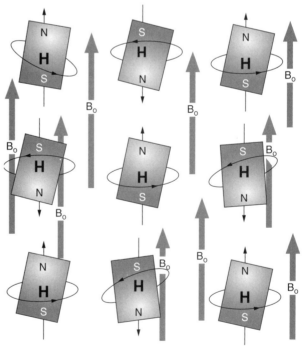

FIG. 1-2 Application of a longitudinal magnetic field (B_o) causes protons to align in a parallel (low energy/α-spin state) and antiparallel (high energy/β-spin state) orientation. The difference in the number of protons in both of these orientations results in a net longitudinal magnetization.

The basis for NMR (nuclear magnetic resonance)/ MRI is the difference between protons in the two different orientations. At rest more protons will be in the parallel than in the anti-parallel orientation, creating a net magnetic moment in the direction of the standing magnetic field. This is the signal that is exploited to create a magnetic resonance image. The greater the strength of the magnet, the greater the difference in energy between protons in the parallel and antiparallel orientations.

When a radiofrequency pulse is applied at the resonant or larmor frequency, energy from the radiofrequency pulse will be absorbed by protons in a low energy orientation, some of which will be moved to a high energy orientation. This will equilibrate the number of protons in the parallel and anti-parallel alignment, creating zero net magnetization along the longitudinal plane. In addition, application of a radiofrequency pulse will cause the protons to spin in a coherent fashion, creating a net transverse magnetization (see Fig. 1-3). A coil placed in the transverse plane (axial plane of the magnet) will have an electrical current induced by the rotating transverse magnetization created in such a fashion. This is the signal measured in MRI and is known as the free

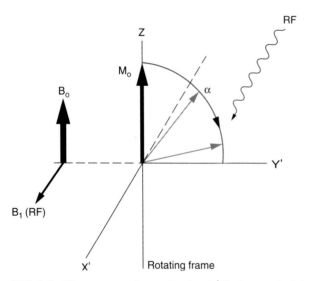

FIG. 1-3   The presence of a standing longitudinal magnetic field (B_o) induces a net longitudinal magnetization (M_o). Application of a radiofrequency pulse (Rf) eliminates the longitudinal magnetization (M_o) by moving protons from a high energy to a low energy state. At the same time, by introducing phase coherence, a net transverse magnetization is created. Application of a radiofrequency pulse is the equivalent of applying a magnetic field in the XY plane (B_1). Application of a radiofrequency pulse will create magnetic signal in the transverse plane (M_{xy}), while reducing the longitudinal magnetic signal. Depending on the length and duration of the radiofrequency pulse, the amount of longitudinal magnetization transferred to the transverse plane can vary. This is represented by the flip angle (α).

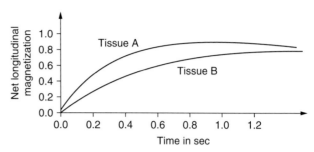

FIG. 1-4   The rate of longitudinal magnetization recovery is described by the T1 time, and can be represented by $M = M_o \times (1 - e^{-(TR/T1)})$. M, the net magnetization; M_0, the original net magnetization; TR, the pulse repetition time in a spin echo pulse sequence; and T1, the spin-lattice relaxation time or longitudinal relaxation time.

induction decay (FID). Protons undergoing FID emit a signal which may be detected and is the basis of MRI. The signal will vary depending upon the density of electrons surrounding the proton.

When the radiofrequency pulse is removed, the longitudinal magnetization will recover, as more protons will return to the parallel rather than the antiparallel state (see Fig. 1-4). The transverse magnetization will decay, as the phase coherence induced by the radiofrequency pulse will dissipate (see Fig. 1-5). The recovery of the longitudinal magnetization of a given tissue is the T1 time (Time to recovery of 66% of the longitudinal magnetization).

The transverse magnetization decay is given by the T2 time (time to loss of 33% of the transverse magnetization signal). T2* refers to the signal loss in the transverse direction from local magnetic field inhomogeneities as well as T2 decay. Different rates of relaxation in the longitudinal (T1) and transverse (T2) directions provide the basis for different types of tissue contrast using different pulse sequences.

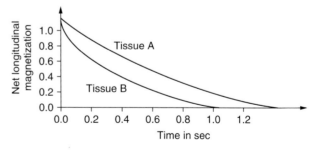

FIG. 1-5   Transverse magnetization decay is described by the T2 time, and is described by the formula $M = M_o \times e^{-(TE/T2)}$. M, the net magnetization; M_0, the original net magnetization; TE, the echo time in a spin echo pulse sequence; and T2, the spin-spin relaxation time or transverse relaxation time.

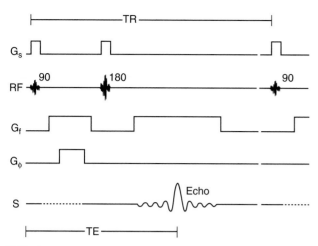

FIG. 1-6 The most basic MRI pulse sequence is a spin echo pulse sequence. A 90 degree and 180 degree pulse are applied while the slice select gradient (G_s) is turned on. Phase encoding (G_p) and frequency encoding gradients (G_f) are applied to provide further spatial localization.

Three orthogonal magnetic gradients are then applied to provide spatial encoding information: a slice select, frequency, and phase encoding (see Fig. 1-6). Parallel imaging techniques replace some of the phase encoding gradients with extra receive coils and thus greatly reduce the amount of time required for imaging.

Gradients create linear variations in the magnetic field strength that protons are exposed to in a given direction. This creates a linear variation in the frequency at which protons precess.

A radiofrequency pulse when applied will have a certain bandwidth, or in other words will cover a range of frequencies. If a gradient is applied along the longitudinal direction, only some protons will precess at the frequencies within the bandwidth of the applied radiofrequency pulse. Thus a finite slice thickness will be excited by the radiofrequency pulse. This is known as a slice select gradient.

After application of the radiofrequency pulse, a second gradient will be applied, known as the phase encoding gradient, along the y-axis. By applying a gradient for a limited period of time, spins will be given spatial information by encoding a different phase dependent on their location (i.e., strength of gradient seen). A final gradient, the frequency encoding gradient, is applied while the transverse magnetization is measured. This gives spins a slightly different precessional frequency dependent on their position along the x-axis.

The application of a radio frequency pulse is used to create an MRI image. Application of a radiofrequency pulse will result in a change in alignment of magnetic spins. Return to the original alignment gives a signal

that can be measured. Different rates of relaxation in the longitudinal (T1) and transverse (T2) directions provide the basis for different types of tissue contrast using different pulse sequences.

The repetition time (TR) is the time between application of a radio frequency pulse. The echo time (TE) is the time of gradient application after application of a radiofrequency pulse to sample the magnetic resonance signal. Having a long TR increases T2 weighting. A short TR increases T1 weighting. A long TE increases T2 weighting. A short TE increases T1 weighting. T1-weighted images have a short TR and TE. T2-weighted images have a long TR and a long TE. Images with a long TR and short TE are proton density-weighted.

Inversion recovery pulses can be used to saturate fat or fluid. In neuroimaging, commonly an inversion recovery pulse is used to eliminate signal from cerebrospinal fluid (CSF). This is called a fluid attenuated inversion recovery (FLAIR) image. Different tissues will have different imaging characteristics based upon composition. Tissues with a short T1 will have bright signal on T1-weighted images. Tissues with a long T2 value will have high signal on T2-weighted images. Bright signal on T1-weighted images is seen with fat, proteinaceous fluid, contrast (gadolinium), blood (in certain stages) and sometimes from the presence of calcium. High T2 signal is most commonly seen in water and in tissue with edema and in gliosis.

Gadolinium administration is used with T1-weighted sequences to take advantage of its paramagnetic effect (T1 shortening) to improve tissue contrast. Gadolinium will delineate blood vessels. Because of the presence of the blood brain barrier, lesions that enhance reflect break down of the blood brain barrier.

MAGNETIC RESONANCE ANGIOGRAPHY

There are multiple effective methods to image the cerebral vasculature using magnetic resonance imaging (see Fig. 1-7). These include time of flight techniques, phase contrast techniques, and contrast enhanced techniques. Time of flight techniques leverage the presence of unsaturated protons in flowing blood to give increased signal in blood vessels compared to background tissue.

Phase contrast **magnetic resonance angiography** (MRA) encodes spins with a different phase shift depending on the velocity at which the spin is moving.

Gadolinium based techniques (contrast enhanced techniques) work because blood vessels have higher contrast agent concentrations than the surrounding tissues.

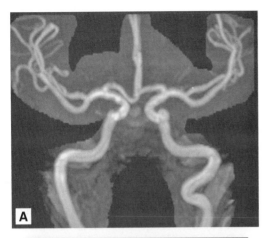

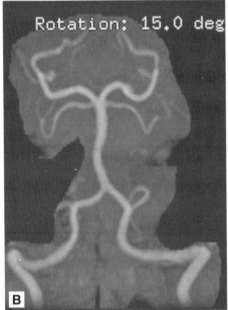

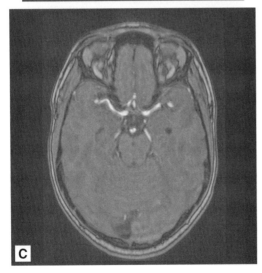

FIG. 1-7 Magnetic resonance angiogram with a time of flight technique can provide high quality maximum intensity projection (MIP) reconstructions of the anterior circulation (A) and the posterior circulation (B) from axial source images (C).

MRI SPECTROSCOPY

MRI spectroscopy is a technique related to conventional MRI. In this technique, chemical shift spectra are generated. The basic techniques are single-voxel and multi-voxel techniques (in which gradients are used to provide spatial information). Important metabolites are lactate, choline, creatine, and *N*-acetyl aspartate (NAA). Lactate is often associated with tissue death. Choline is a marker for cell turnover, with elevated levels reflecting increased turnover, commonly associated with malignancies. Creatine is an internal reference. NAA is a marker found in normal neuronal tissue.

MRI PERFUSION

MRI perfusion is a new technique used in the evaluation of tumors and strokes. Gadolinium circulation through the brain is tracked through its first pass through the circulation. At this concentration, gadolinium has a T2 shortening effect. This can be used to measure cerebral blood flow, blood volume, and mean transit time, values that are useful in the evaluation of stroke and tumor patients.

DIFFUSION WEIGHTED IMAGING

Diffusion weighted imaging measures random Brownian microscopic particle movement. In an ischemic stroke, cell death results in failure of the Na/K ATPase, resulting in intracellular swelling and thus restricted diffusion. Some cellular tumors and intracranial abscesses also can have restricted diffusion.

MRI VENOGRAPHY

MRI venography is a collection of techniques for visualizing the venous system. Phase contrast techniques, time of flight techniques, or contrast enhanced techniques may be used.

BASICS OF CT PHYSICS

Computed axial tomography (CT), introduced by Sir Godfrey Hounsfield in the early 1970s, utilizes x-ray tubes and detectors to create a cross-sectional image of a defined slice thickness. Attenuation values in each pixel are reconstructed by mathematical means (filtered back projection).

These attenuation values are displayed as Hounsfield units, with water being held as the standard zero value.

The typical range of Hounsfield units is from −1000 to 1000. Water measures by definition as zero Hounsfield units, air as −1000.

Early scanners acquired one slice at a time. The development of slip ring technology allowed the development of spiral or helical CT scanning. In this type of system, the patient table moves while the x-ray tube makes a rotation to acquire 3D volumetric data.

The latest scanners combine helical technology with multiple detectors. This has improved scanning speeds (and subsequent improved temporal resolution resulting in fewer motion artifacts), scan coverage, and resolution. Isotropic voxel acquisition is now possible.

These developments have led to great improvements in techniques of vascular imaging with CT, such as CT angiography and venography, as well as improved the three-dimensional reconstruction capabilities for definition of bony anatomy. Dynamic contrast enhanced CT scans can be used to measure cerebral blood flow, cerebral blood volume, and mean transit time for the evaluation of ischemia.

REFERENCES

Hashemi RH, Bradley WG. *MRI: The Basics*. Baltimore, MD: Williams and Wilkins; 1997.

Liney G. *MRI in Clinical Practice*. London: Springer-Verlag; 2006.

Mahadevappa M. The AAPM/RSNA physics tutorial for residents. Search for isotropic resolution in CT from conventional through multiple-row detector. *Radiographics*. 2002;22:949–62.

Rydberg J, Buckwalter KA, Caldemeyer KS, et al. Multi-section CT: scanning techniques and clinical applications. *Radiographics*. 2000;20:1787–1806.

Chapter 2

NEUROANATOMY BASICS

A basic working knowledge of neuroanatomy is necessary to interpret neuroimaging studies.

CELLULAR ANATOMY

Neurons and glial cells are the basic cellular units of the nervous system (see Fig. 2-1). Neurons are the functional units, while glial cells provide structural and metabolic support. Neurons are composed of axons, dendrites, and soma. Dendrites receive electrical signals from other neurons. Axons conduct electrical signals away from the cell to the synapse. The cell body or soma contains the nucleus and other organelles.

NERVOUS SYSTEM

The nervous system is divided into the peripheral nervous system (PNS) and the central nervous system (CNS).

PERIPHERAL NERVOUS SYSTEM

The PNS has somatic and autonomic divisions (see Fig. 2-2). There are 31 pairs of spinal nerves: 8 cervical, 12 thoracic, 5 lumbar, 5 sacral, and 1 coccygeal. Spinal nerves contain motor and sensory fibers, and have muscular and cutaneous branches.

AUTONOMIC NERVES
The autonomic nervous system implements hypothalamic and brainstem control of body functions (see Fig. 2-3).

SYMPATHETIC NERVES
Preganglionic neuron cell bodies are in the thoracic and upper lumbar spine. The sympathetic nervous system mediates the fight or flight response. Postganglionic neurons are found distant from target organs in paravertebral ganglia.

PARASYMPATHETIC NERVES
The parasympathetic system conserves energy. Preganglionic neurons are in the CNS or sacrum. Post ganglionic neurons are found close to the target organ.

CENTRAL NERVOUS SYSTEM

The CNS is composed of the spinal cord and brain.

SPINE
The spinal cord extends from the skull base to approximately the level of L2. The caudal end of the spinal cord is known as the conus medullaris. The cauda equina starts at the terminal end of the conus and contains the lumbar and sacral nerve roots. If the conus medullaris lies below L2/3 intervertebral disk level, there is concern for cord tethering.

The spinal canal contains central grey matter, in a butterfly shape, composed of dorsal and ventral horns (see Fig. 2-4). The dorsal horn is a receptive sensory region. The ventral horn is the motor region. The central canal is a component of the ventricular system. Somatic sensory receptor neurons enter through the dorsal root ganglion.

The peripheral white matter of the spinal cord contains both ascending (sensory) and descending (motor) tracts.

The two major sensory systems are the dorsal column/medial lemniscus (proprioception) pathway and the anterolateral system (pain and temperature). The anterolateral system is composed of the spinothalamic tracts, which cross to the contralateral side of the spinal cord within 1–2 segments of entering the cord.

The major descending white matter pathways include the corticospinal, rubrospinal, vestibulospinal, reticulospinal, and tectospinal tracts.

The dermatomes of the body have a segmental organization (see Fig. 2-5).

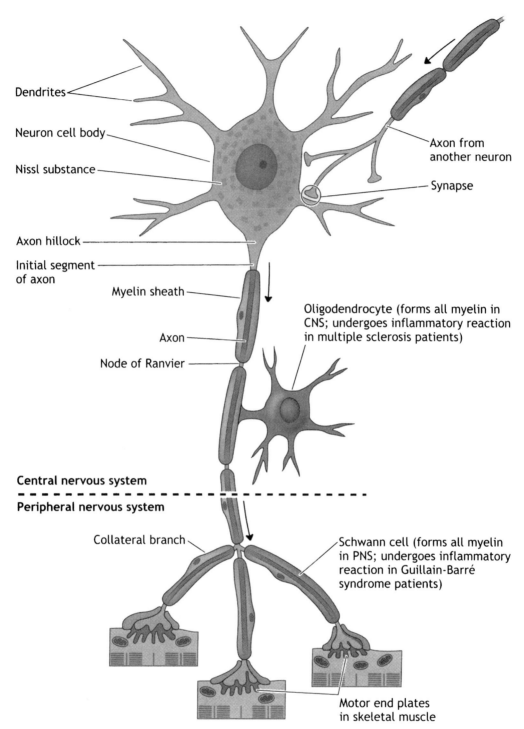

FIG. 2-1 Features of a skeletal motor neuron.
SOURCE: White JS. *USMLE Road Map Neuroscience*. Lange Medical Books/McGraw Hill; 2002.

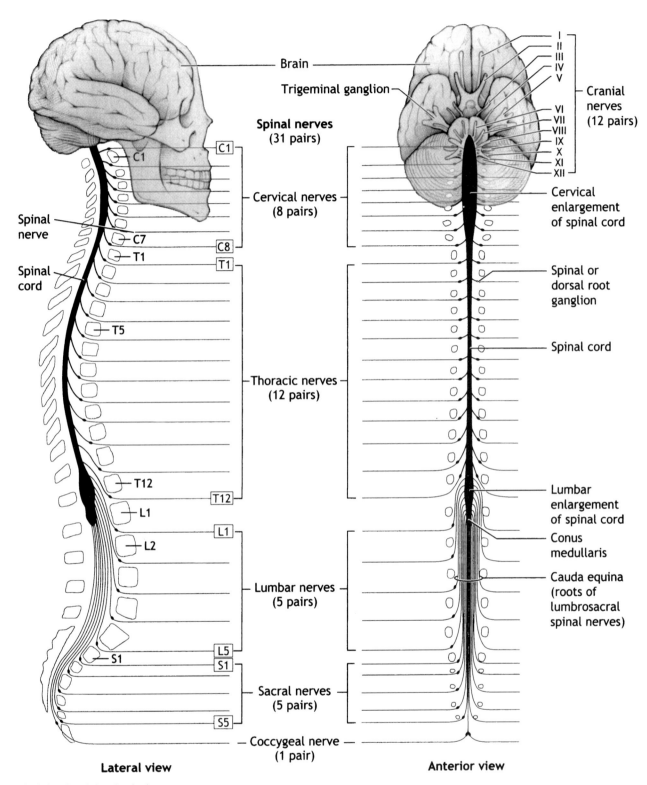

Lateral view

Anterior view

Brain

Trigeminal ganglion

Spinal nerves
(31 pairs)

Cranial
nerves
(12 pairs)

I
II
III
IV
V
VI
VII
VIII
IX
X
XI
XII

Cervical
enlargement
of spinal cord

Cervical nerves
(8 pairs)

Spinal or
dorsal root
ganglion

Spinal cord

Thoracic nerves
(12 pairs)

Lumbar
enlargement
of spinal cord

Conus
medullaris

Lumbar nerves
(5 pairs)

Cauda equina
(roots of
lumbrosacral
spinal nerves)

Sacral nerves
(5 pairs)

Coccygeal nerve
(1 pair)

Spinal
nerve

Spinal
cord

C1

C7
C8
T1

T5

T12

L1

L2

S1

C1

T1

T12

L1

L5
S1

S5

FIG. 2-2 Cranial and spinal nerves.

Source: White JS. *USMLE Road Map Neuroscience.* Lange Medical Books/McGraw Hill; 2002.

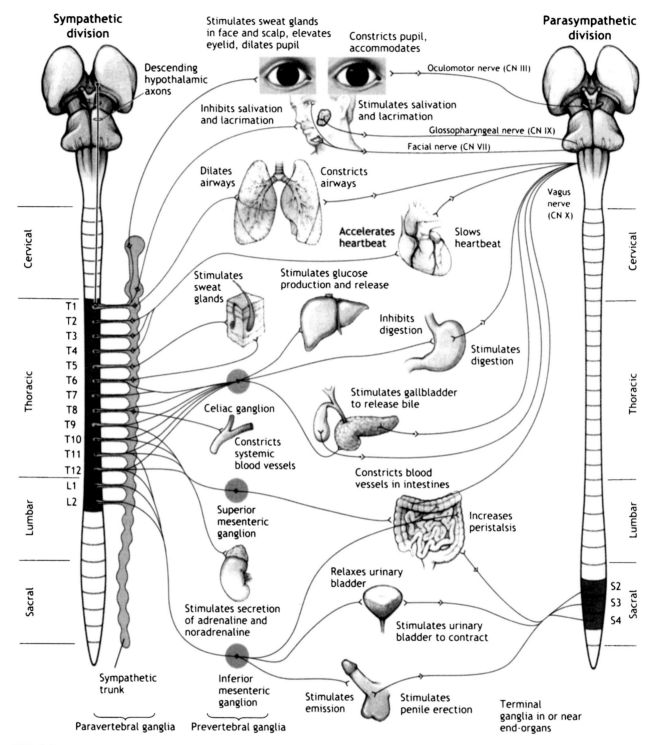

FIG. 2-3   Autonomic nerves.
Source: White JS. *USMLE Road Map Neuroscience.* Lange Medical Books/McGraw Hill; 2002.

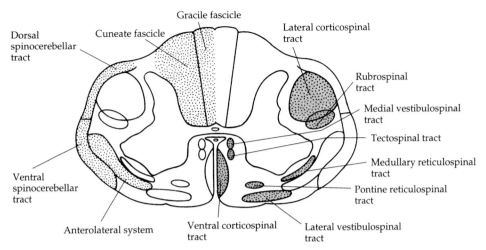

FIG. 2-4 Schematic diagram of the spinal cord, indicating the locations of the ascending (*left*) and descending (*right*) pathways.
Source: Martin JH. *Neuroanatomy Text and Atlas*. The McGraw Hill Companies; 2003.

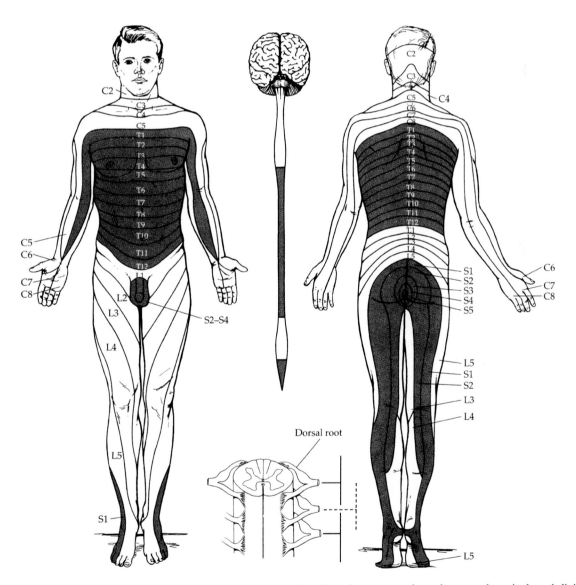

FIG. 2-5 The dermatomes of the body have a segmental organization. Note the correspondence between the spinal cord divisions (Shown on a ventral view of the central nervous system) and dermatome locations.
Source: Martin JH. *Neuroanatomy Text and Atlas*. The McGraw Hill Companies; 2003. Figure 5-4, page 116.

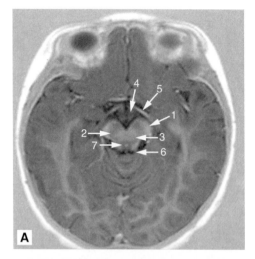

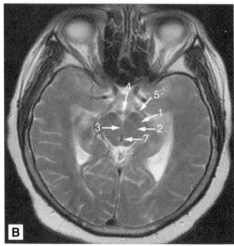

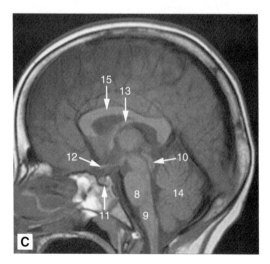

FIG. 2-6 Axial and sagittal MRI scans depict the normal anatomy of the brainstem.
1. Cerebral peduncle   2. Substantia nigra   3. Red nucleus   4. Mamillary body   5. Optic tract   6. Superior colliculus   7. Central canal   8. Pons   9. Medulla   10. Tectum-superior and inferior colliculi   11. Pituitary gland   12. Optic chiasm   13. Fornix   14. Cerebellum   15. Corpus callosum

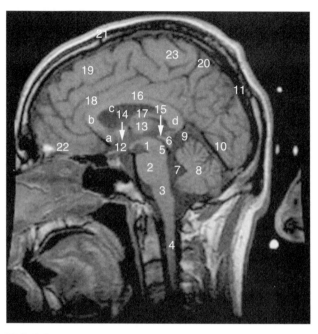

FIG. 2-7 Normal anatomy seen on a midline sagittal MRI scan. 1. Midbrain   2. Pons   3. Medulla oblongata   4. Spinal cord   5. Aqueduct of sylvius   6. Quadrigeminal plate   7. IV ventricle   8. Cerebellum   9. Vein of Galen   10. Straight sinus   11. Superior sagittal sinus   12. III ventricle   13. Massa intermedia   14. Anterior commissure   15. Posterior commissure   16. Corpus callosum : a. Rostrum b. Genu c. Body d. Splenium   17. Fornix   18. Cingulate gyrus   19. Superior frontal gyrus   20. Sulcus of Rolandus   21. Coronal suture   22. Orbitofrontal cortex   23. Paracentral lobule.

BRAINSTEM

The brainstem is composed of the midbrain, pons, and medulla. The major structures in each are listed below:

- Midbrain:
  - Cranial nerves III and IV arise from the medulla.
  - Tectum:
    - Superior colliculi-conjugate gaze
    - Inferior colliculi-auditory structures
  - The cerebral peduncles and substantia nigra
  - Interpeduncular fossa
  - The cerebral aqueduct
- Pons:
  - Cranial nerves V, VI, VII, VIII
- Medulla:
  - Cranial nerves IX, X, and XII
  - Pyramidal decussation

The MRI appearance of the midbrain and brainstem are shown in Fig. 2-6. Figure 2-7 details the normal anatomy seen on a midline sagittal MRI scan.

CRANIAL NERVES

The cranial nerves are organized into three major columns (see Fig. 2-8 and Table 2-1)):

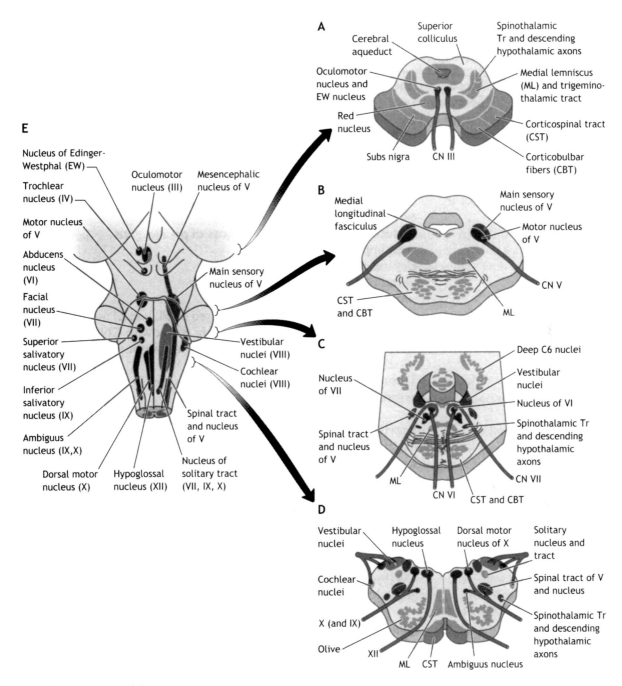

FIG. 2-8 Cranial nerve nuclei.
SOURCE: White JS. *USMLE Road Map Neuroscience.* Lange Medical Books/McGraw Hill; 2002.

TABLE 2-1 The cranial nerves

CRANIAL NERVE AND ROOT	FUNCTION	CRANIAL FORAMINA	PERIPHERAL SENSORY GANGLIA	CNS NUCLEUS	PERIPHERAL AUTONOMIC GANGLIA	PERIPHERAL STRUCTURE INNERVATED
I Olfactory	Smell	Cribriform plate		Olfactory bulb		Olfactory receptors of olfactory epithelium
II Optic	Vision	Optic		Lateral geniculate nucleus		Retina (ganglion cells)
III Oculomotor	Somatic skeletal motor	Superior orbital fissure		Oculomotor		Medial, superior, inferior, rectus, inferior oblique, and levator palpebrae muscles
	Autonomic			Edinger-Westphal	Ciliary	Constrictor muscles of iris, ciliary muscle
IV Trochlear	Somatic skeletal motor	Superior orbital fissure		Trochlear		Superior oblique muscle
V Trigeminal	Somatic sensory	Superior orbital fissure (Ophthalmic)	Semilunar	Spinal nucleus, main sensory nucleus, mesencephalic nucleus of CN V		Skin and mucous membranes of the head, muscle receptors, meninges
		Rotundum (Maxillary)				
	Branchiomeric motor	Ovale (Mandibular)		Motor nucleus of CN V		Jaw muscles, tensor tympani, tensor palati, and digastric (anterior belly)
VI Abducens	Somatic skeletal motor	Superior orbital fissure		Abducens		Lateral rectus muscle
VII Intermediate	Taste	Internal auditory meatus	Geniculate	Solitary nucleus		Taste (anterior two-thirds of tongue), palate
	Somatic sensory	Internal auditory meatus	Geniculate	Spinal nucleus of CN V		Skin of external ear
	Autonomic			Superior salivatory	Pterygopalatine, submandibular	Lacrimal glands, glands of nasal mucosa, salivary glands
Facial	Branchiomeric motor	Internal auditory meatus		Facial		Muscles of facial expression, digastric (posterior belly), and stapedius
VIII Vestibulocochlear	Hearing	Internal auditory meatus	Spiral	Cochlear		Hair cells in organ of Corti
	Balance		Vestibular	Vestibular		Hair cells in vestibular labyrinth

CN	Name	Functional component	Ganglion	Nucleus		Innervation / Target
IX	Glossopharyngeal	Somatic sensory	Jugular	Spinal nucleus of CN V		Skin of external ear
		Viscerosensory	Superior Petrosal (inferior)	Solitary nucleus (caudal)		Mucous membranes in pharyngeal region, middle ear, carotid body, and sinus
		Taste	Petrosal	Solitary nucleus (rostral)		Taste (posterior one-third of tongue)
		Autonomic		Inferior salivatory nucleus	Otic	Parotid gland
		Branchiomeric motor		Ambiguus (rostral)		Striated muscles of pharynx
X	Vagus	Somatic sensory	Jugular	Spinal nucleus of CN V		Skin of external ear, meninges
		Viscerosensory	Nodose (inferior)	Solitary nucleus (caudal)		Larynx, trachea, gut, aortic arch receptors
		Taste	Nodose (inferior)	Solitary nucleus (rostral)		Taste buds (posterior oral cavity, larynx)
		Autonomic		Dorsal motor nucleus of CN X	Peripheral autonomic	Gut (to splenic flexure of colon), respiratory structures, heart
		Branchiomeric motor		Ambiguus (middle region)		Striated muscles of palate pharynx, and larynx
XI	Spinal accessory	Branchiomeric motor	Jugular	Ambiguus (caudal)		Striated muscles of larynx (Aberrant vague branches)
		Unclassified[1]	Jugular	Accesory nucleus, pyramidal decussation of C3–C5		sternocleidomastoid and portion of trapezius muscles
XII	Hypoglossal	Somatic skeletal motor	Hypoglossal	Hypoglossal[1]		Intrinsic muscles of tongue, hyoglossus, genioglossus, and styloglossus muscles

Abbreviation key: CN, cranial nerve.

[1] The accessory nucleus is unclassified because some of the muscles (or compartments of muscles) innervated by this nucleus develop from the occipital somites.

SOURCE: Martin JH. *Neuroanatomy Text and Atlas.* The McGraw Hill Companies; 2003.

1. Somatic motor nuclei (innervates striated muscle derived from occipital somites), including tongue and extraocular muscles (CN III, IV, VI, XII)

2. Brachiomotor column (supplies derivatives of the branchial arches) which includes CN V motor nucleus, CN VII nucleus, and CN XI

3. Visceromotor column or autonomic motor column comprises the parasympathetic nervous system, CN III (nucleus of Edinger-Westphal), CN VII (superior salivatory nucleus), CN IX (inferior salivatory nucleus), and dorsal motor nucleus of the facial nerve

MENINGEAL LAYERS

There are three primary meningeal layers.

1. Dura: Thick outer layer with a protective function. Outer periosteal and inner meningeal layer. Falx cerebri and tentorium cerebelli.

2. Arachnoid: Has potential space—the subdural space between dura and arachnoid.

3. Pia: Innermost layer—between pia and arachnoid is the subarachnoid space.

CEREBELLUM

The cerebellum is involved in planning and fine tuning movement. The cerebellum influences contralateral motor neurons in the cerebral cortex and brainstem.

DIENCEPHALON

The diencephalon consists of the thalamus and the hypothalamus.

Thalamus: The thalamus is a relay center for motor and sensory nuclei (see Fig. 2-9).

Hypothalamus: The hypothalamus maintains homeostasis through interactions with the pituitary gland and limbic system.

BRAIN

SURFACE ANATOMY

The brain is divided into frontal, temporal, parietal, and occipital regions (see Fig. 2-10). The frontal lobe and parietal lobe are divided by the central sulcus. The frontal lobe contains the motor cortex, the premotor cortex, and the prefrontal cortex.

Broca's speech area (nonfluent aphasia) is also located along the inferior aspect of the frontal lobe (dominant hemisphere, usually left). The parietal lobe contains the primary somatosensory cortex as well as the somatosensory association cortex. The occipital lobe contains the primary and visual association cortices.

The temporal lobe contains the primary auditory cortex (Heschl's gyrus), Wernicke's (fluent aphasia) speech area on the dominant hemisphere, and the limbic system (hippocampus and amygdala). The hippocampal formation is involved with memory consolidation. The efferent pathway of the hippocampus is the fornix. This terminates in the mamillary bodies.

The frontal and parietal lobes are divided by the central sulcus. There are two primary ways to identify the central sulcus on MRI. The superior frontal sulcus intersects the prefrontal sulcus. The next most posterior sulcus is the central sulcus (see Fig. 2-11). On sagittal images, the central sulcus is the first sulcus in front of the ascending ramus of the cingulate sulcus. The motor cortex has a somatotopic organization (see Fig. 2-12).

The basal ganglia are involved in the initiation of movement, and are divided into the caudate, putamen, and globus pallidus (see Fig. 2-13).

The posterior limb of the internal capsule contains motor fibers from descending white matter tracts.

VENTRICLES

Cerebrospinal fluid (CSF) protects the brain from physical shocks and acts as a medium for chemical communications. CSF is produced primarily in the choroid

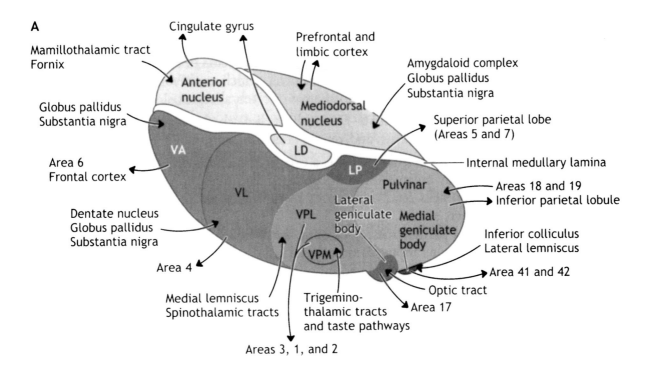

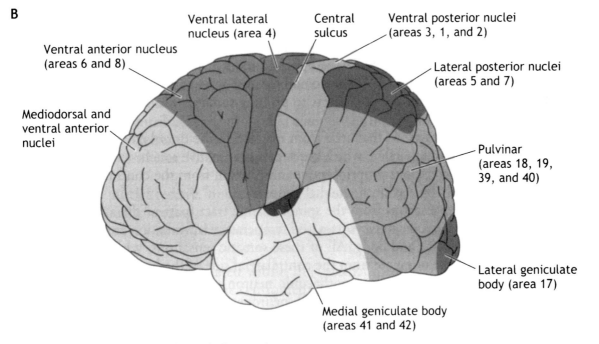

FIG. 2-9   A and **B.** The thalamus and its cortical connections.
SOURCE: White JS. *USMLE Road Map Neuroscience.* Lange Medical Books/McGraw Hill; 2002.

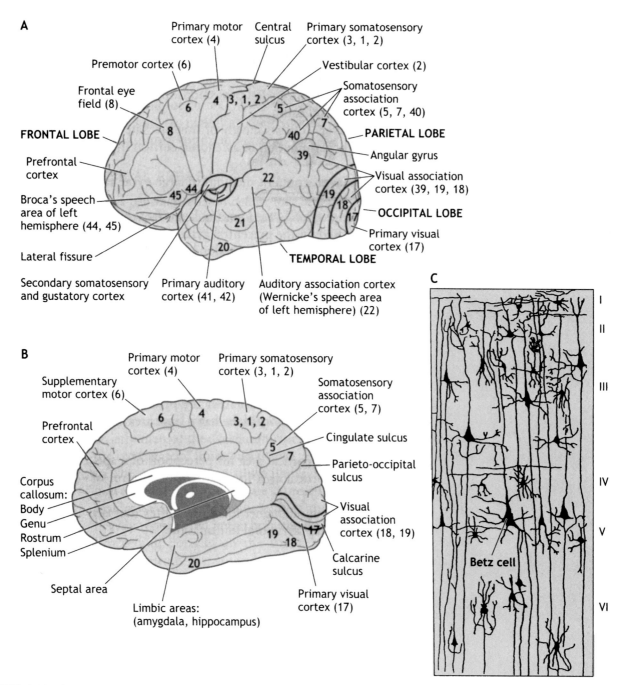

FIG. 2-10 **A** and **B.** Motor and sensory areas of the cerebral cortex. **C.** Cortical layers.
Source: White JS. *USMLE Road Map Neuroscience.* Lange Medical Books/McGraw Hill; 2002.

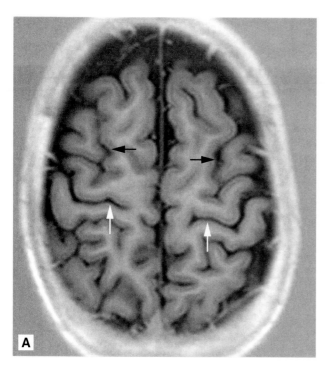
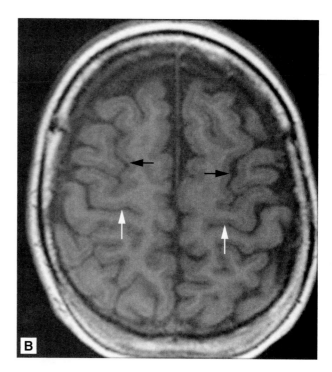
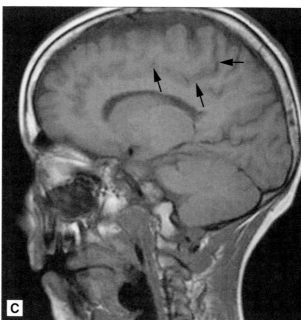

FIG. 2-11 **A** and **B.** The superior frontal sulcus (black arrows) intersects the prefrontal sulcus. The central sulcus (white arrows) is the sulcus behind the prefrontal sulcus. **C.** The ascending ramus of the cingulate sulcus (black arrows) can also be used to identify the central sulcus. The central sulcus is immediately anterior to the ascending ramus of the cingulate sulcus.

A

Motor homunculus
(precentral gyrus)

Sensory homunculus
(postcentral gyrus)

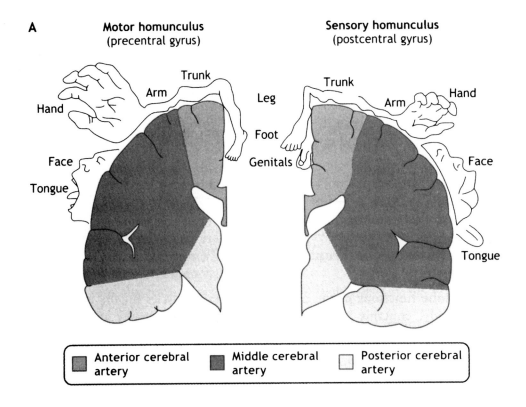

Anterior cerebral artery ▮   Middle cerebral artery ▮   Posterior cerebral artery □

B

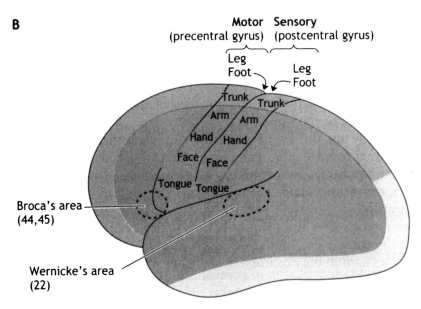

FIG. 2-12 A. Arterial supply and homunculi of primary motor and sensory cortex (coronal view). **B.** Arterial supply of primary motor and sensory cortex (lateral view). Note the motor cortex has a somatotopic organization (see Fig. 2-10).
SOURCE: Homonculus: White JS. *USMLE Road Map Neuroscience.* Lange Medical Books/McGraw Hill; 2002.

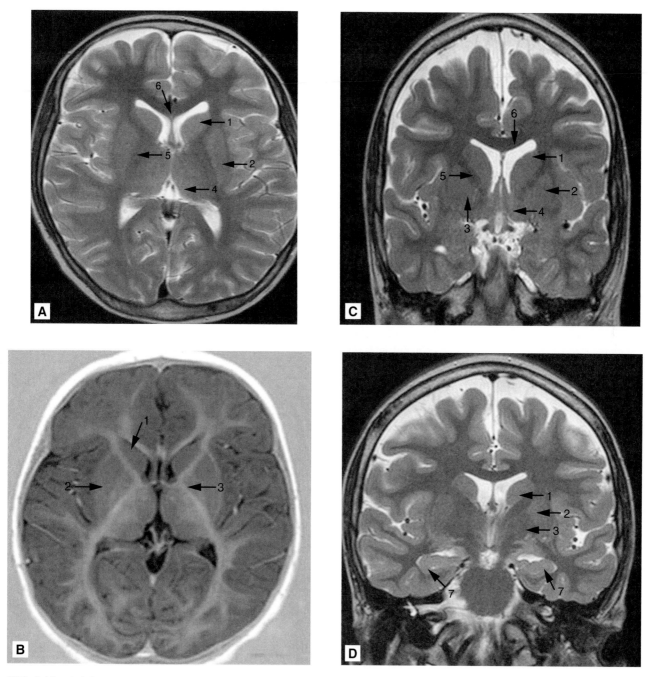

FIG. 2-13   Axial and coronal MR images of the basal ganglia and surrounding structures.
1. Caudate 2. Putamen 3. Globus pallidus 4. Thalamus 5. Internal capsule 6. Corpus callosum 7. Hippocampus.

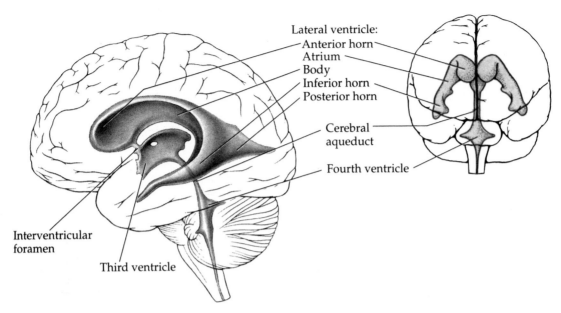

FIG. 2-14 Ventricular system. The lateral ventricle, third ventricle, cerebral aqueduct, and fourth ventricle are seen from the lateral brain surface (left) and the front (right). The lateral ventricle is divided into four main components: anterior (or frontal) horn, body, inferior (or temporal) horn, and the posterior (or occipital) horn. The interventricular foramen (of Monro) connects each lateral ventricle with the third ventricle. The cerebral aqueduct connects the third and fourth ventricles.
SOURCE: Martin JH. *Neuroanatomy Text and Atlas.* The McGraw Hill Companies; 2003. Figure 1-11, page 19.

plexus. The choroid plexus is found in the body and inferior horn of the lateral ventricles, in the third, and fourth ventricles. About 400–500 mL is produced daily. The average adult has 90–150 mL of CSF.

The lateral ventricles have a body, anterior (frontal), inferior (temporal), and posterior (occipital) horns. They have a confluence called the atrium. The intraventricular foramen of Munro connects the lateral ventricles to the third ventricle (see Fig. 2-14). The third ventricle drains through the cerebral aqueduct of Sylvius into the fourth ventricle. The outflow of the fourth ventricle is through the foramina of Magendie and Luschka.

VENOUS ANATOMY

The normal venous drainage of the brain is divided into superficial and deep veins (see Fig. 2-15). Both venous systems drain into the dural venous sinuses. The dominant superficial cortical draining vein into the superior sagittal sinus is known as the vein of Trolard. The dominant superficial vein draining into the lateral sinus is the vein of Labbe.

The deep cerebral venous drainage system consists of the internal cerebral veins (composed of the anterior septal and thalamostriate veins) and the basal veins of Rosenthal. These veins join to form the vein of Galen. The junction of the vein of Galen with the inferior sagittal sinus forms the straight sinus.

The superior sagittal sinus and straight sinus form the torcula. They then drain into the transverse sinuses, which in turn drain into the sigmoid sinus which drains into the jugular vein. This provides the vast majority of the venous drainage pathway for the brain.

ARTERIAL ANATOMY

The arterial supply to the brain is provided by two internal carotid arteries and two vertebral arteries (see Fig. 2-16). Each internal carotid artery bifurcates into a middle cerebral artery (MCA) and anterior cerebral artery (ACA).

The internal carotid artery contains the cervical, petrous, lacerum, cavernous, clinoid, opthalmic, and communicating segments.

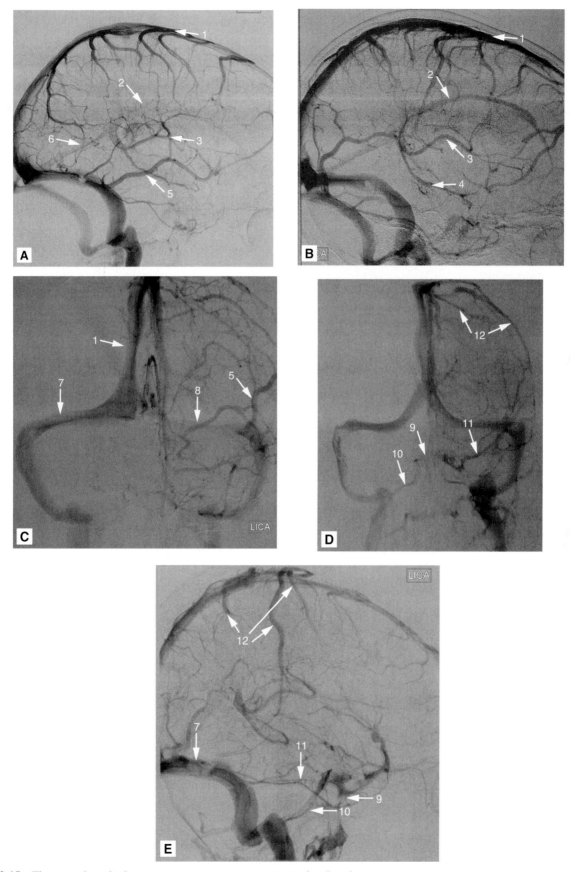

FIG. 2-15 The normal cerebral venous anatomy as seen on a conventional angiogram.
1. Superior sagittal sinus   2. Inferior sagittal sinus   3. Internal cerebral vein   4. Basal vein of Rosenthal   5. Vein of Labbe   6. Straight sinus 7. Right transverse sinus   8. Left transverse sinus   9. Cavernous sinus   10. Inferior petrosal sinus   11. Superior petrosal sinus 12. Cortical superficial draining veins.

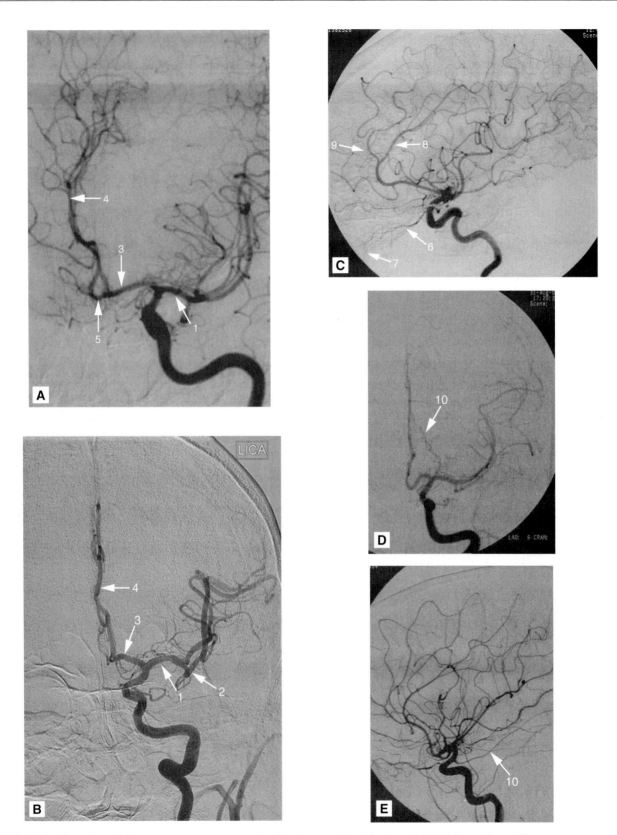

FIG. 2-16   Normal arterial anatomy seen on a conventional angiogram after injection of the left internal carotid artery.
1. Middle cerebral artery (M1)   2. Middle cerebral artery bifurcation   3. Anterior cerebral artery (A1)   4. Anterior cerebral artery (A2)
5. Anterior communicating artery   6. Opthalmic artery   7. Choroidal blush   8. Pericallosal artery   9. Callosomarginal artery
10. Posterior communicating artery.

Important branches include the ophthalmic, anterior choroidal, and posterior communicating arteries.

The anterior choroidal artery supplies the globus pallidus, genu, and posterior limb of the internal capsule, as well as the medial temporal lobe.

The MCA divides into a superior and inferior division. The superior division supplies the lateral frontal lobe and anterior parietal lobe. The inferior division supplies the superior temporal lobe and posterior parietal lobe. The MCA has small perforating branches, the lenticulostriate arteries, which supply the body of the caudate and the putamen.

The ACA supplies the medial and inferior frontal lobe and medial parietal lobe. Common anatomic variants include unilateral hypoplasia of an A1 segment or a combined A2 segment of the ACA.

Small perforating branches, the medial lenticulostriate, supply the anterior limb of the internal capsule and the head of the caudate.

The posterior circulation is supplied by the paired vertebral arteries, which form the basilar artery (see Fig. 2-17).

The vertebral arteries give off a posterior inferior cerebellar artery (PICA) before uniting to form the basilar artery.

The basilar artery terminates in the posterior cerebral arteries.

The other branches of the basilar artery include the superior cerebellar artery (SCA) and the anterior inferior cerebellar artery (AICA). Common variants include a common AICA/PICA trunk, a duplicated SCA or AICA, an extradural or low origin of the PICA. Usually one vertebral

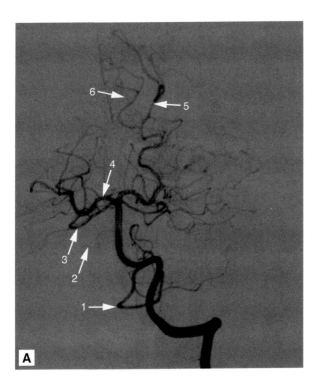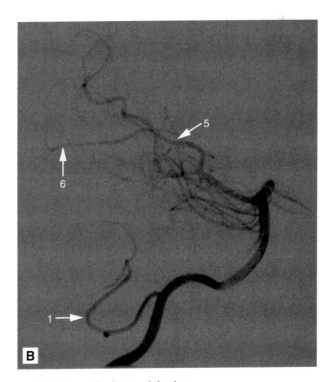

FIG. 2-17 Normal arterial anatomy seen on a conventional angiogram after left vertebral artery injection.
1. Posterior inferior cerebellar artery   2. Anterior inferior cerebellar artery   3. Superior cerebellar artery   4. Posterior cerebral artery
5. Parietal branches of posterior cerebral artery   6. Occipital/Calcarine branches of posterior cerebral artery.

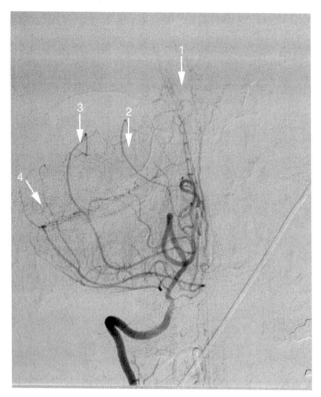

FIG. 2-18 AP view from a conventional angiogram with selective injection of a right vertebral artery that ends in a posterior inferior cerebellar artery.
1. Vermian branches   2. Median hemispheric branches
3. Interhemispheric branches   4. Lateral hemispheric branches

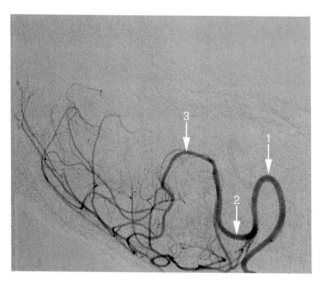

FIG. 2-19 Lateral view from a conventional angiogram with selective injection of a right vertebral artery that ends in a posterior inferior cerebellar artery.
1. Anterior and lateral medullary   2. Tonsillomedullary segment
3. Televeotonsillar segment

artery is dominant, most commonly the left. The course of the PICA is given below (see Figs. 2-18 and 2-19).

SPINAL CORD ARTERIAL ANATOMY SUPPLY

The primary blood supply to the spinal cord is from the anterior spinal artery and the paired posterior spinal arteries.

The anterior spinal artery is formed by the junction of feeders from both vertebral arteries, and is reinforced by segmental feeders. These can come from the vertebral artery, thyrocervical, or costocervical trunk, and intercostal arteries at the thoracic and lumbar levels.

The largest segmental feeder is the artery of Adamkiewicz, which usually arises in the thoracic spine on the left side between T8 and T12 (85%). There can be a dominant thoracic feeder between T5-T8 (artery of Lazorthes) (see Fig. 2-20).

The paired posterior spinal arteries can rarely be seen angiographically.

VISUAL SYSTEM

Visual signals are detected by the retina, then nerve impulses are conducted by the optic nerve to the optic chiasm. At the optic chiasm, the medial fibers (representing the temporal visual fields) cross (see Fig. 2-21).

After the optic chiasm, the optic tracts project to the lateral geniculate nucleus of the thalamus, the hypothalamus (controls Circadian rhythms), the pretectal nucleus (controls pupillary reflexes through III rd nerve and Edinger-Westphal nuclei), and the superior colliculus (controls conjugate gaze).

The output of the lateral geniculate nucleus is through the optic radiations (see Fig. 2-22).

MOTOR PATHWAY OVERVIEW

There are many pathways involved in the control of movement. The cerebral cortex and brainstem contribute to descending motor pathways. The basal ganglia and cerebellum play an important regulatory role. The cerebellum is involved in planning and fine-tuning of movements. The basal ganglia are involved in the initiation of movement.

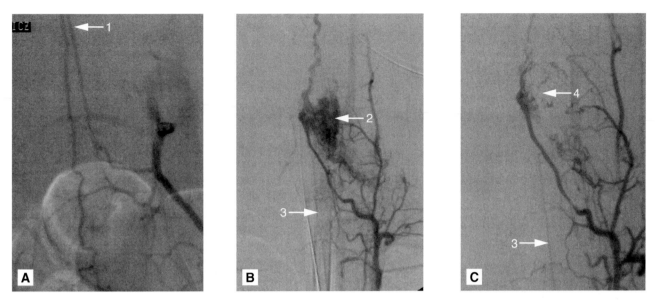

FIG. 2-20 Normal arterial supply to the anterior spinal artery includes the artery of Adamkiewicz and the artery of Lazorthes.
1. Classic hairpin loop of the artery of Adamkiewicz with selective injection of the T11 intercostal artery.   2. Large spine arteriovenous fistula supplied by an enlarged thoracic feeding artery.   3. Anterior spinal artery arising from a dominant thoracic intercostal feeder (T5), also known as the artery of Lazorthes.   4. Post embolization images of the arteriovenous fistula arising from the artery of Lazorthes. (Courtesy of Victor Aletieh, MD.)

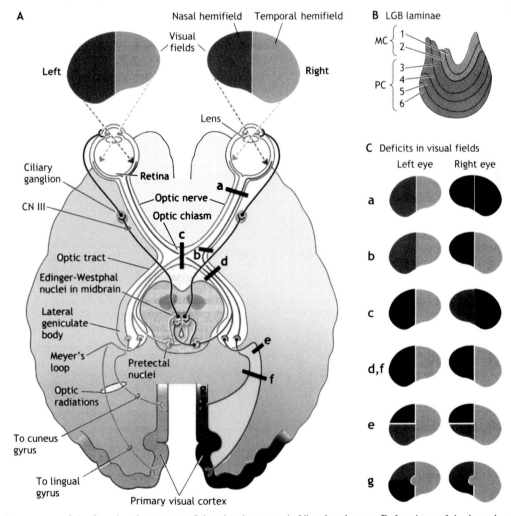

FIG. 2-21 A summary of the functional anatomy of the visual system **A.** Visual pathways. **B.** Laminae of the lateral geniculate body. **C.** Common visual field deficits.
SOURCE: White JS. *USMLE Road Map Neuroscience.* Lange Medical Books/McGraw Hill; 2002.

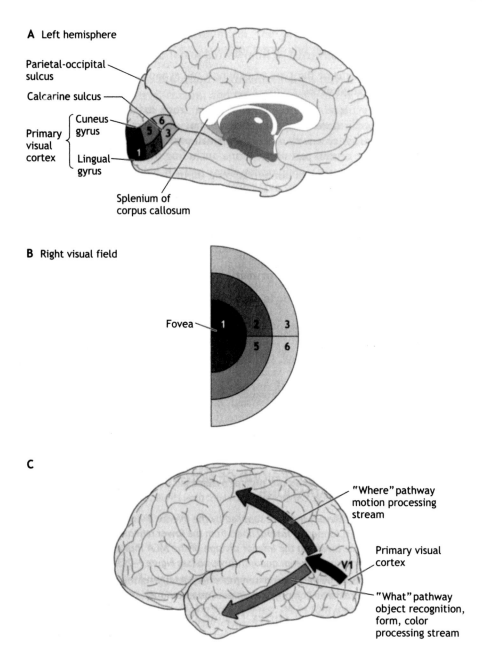

A Left hemisphere

Parietal-occipital sulcus

Calcarine sulcus

Cuneus gyrus

Primary visual cortex

Lingual gyrus

Splenium of corpus callosum

B Right visual field

Fovea

C

"Where" pathway motion processing stream

Primary visual cortex

V1

"What" pathway object recognition, form, color processing stream

FIG. 2.22   A, B, and **C.** Cortical representation of visual field and cortical processing streams.
SOURCE: White JS. *USMLE Road Map Neuroscience.* Lange Medical Books/McGraw Hill; 2002.

The limbic and prefrontal motor areas are important in the decision to make a movement. The premotor area is important in forming a motor plan of action (see Fig. 2-23).

The major descending pathways are the lateral corticospinal tract, the anterior corticospinal tract, the corticobulbar tract (all of which originate in the cerebral cortex), and from the brainstem: the rubrospinal, reticulospinal, tectospinal, and vestibulospinal tracts. Fibers of the lateral corticospinal tract and rubrospinal tract decussate (see Table 2-2 and Fig. 2-24).

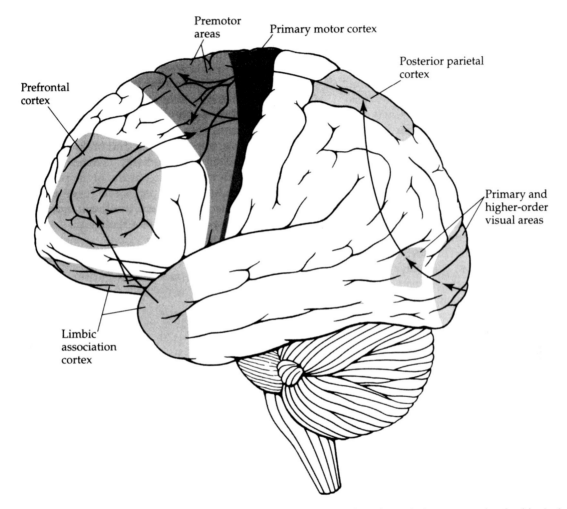

FIG. 2-23 Key cortical regions for controlling movement. The limbic and prefrontal association areas are involved in the initial decision to move, in relation to motivational and emotional factors. In reaching to grasp an object, the visual areas process information about the location and shape of the object. This information is transmitted, via the posterior parietal lobe, to the premotor areas, which are important in movement planning. From there, information is transmitted to the primary motor cortex, from which descending control signals are sent to the motor neurons.
SOURCE: Martin JH. *Neuroanatomy Text and Atlas.* The McGraw Hill Companies; 2003.

TABLE 2-2. Descending pathways for controlling movement

TRACT	SITE OF ORIGIN	DECUSSATION	SPINAL CORD COLUMN	SITE OF TERMINATION	FUNCTION
Cerebral Cortex					
Corticospinal					
Lateral	Areas 6, 4, 1, 2, 3, 5, 7, 23	Crossed—pyramidal decussation	Lateral	Dorsal horn, lateral intermediate zone, ventral horn	Sensory control, voluntary movement (limb muscles)
Ventral	Areas 6, 4	Uncrossed[3]	Ventral	Medial intermediate zone, ventral horn	Voluntary movement (axial muscles)
Corticobulbar	Areas 6, 4, 1, 2, 3, 5, 7, 23	Crossed and uncrossed[2]	Brain stem only	Cranial nerve sensory and motor nuclei, reticular formation	Sensory control, voluntary movement (cranial muscles)
Brain Stem					
Rubrospinal	Red nucleus (magnocellular)	Ventral tegmentum	Lateral	Lateral intermediate zone, ventral horn	Voluntary movement, limb muscles
Vestibulospinal Lateral	Lateral Vestibular Nucleus	Ipsilateral[1]	Ventral	Medical intermediate zone, ventral horn	Balance
Medial	Medial vestibular nucleus	Bilateral	Ventral	Medial intermediate zone, ventral horn	Head position/neck muscles
Reticulospinal Pontine	Pontine reticular formation	Ipsilateral[1]	Ventral	Medial intermediate horn, ventral horn	Autonomic movement, axial and limb muscles
Medullary	Medullary reticular formation	Ipsilateral[1]	Ventrolateral	Medial Intermediate zone, ventral horn	Autonomic movement, axial and limb muscles
Tectospinal	Deep superior colliculus	Dorsal tegmentum	Ventral	Medial intermediate zone, ventral horn	Coordinates neck with eye movements

[1]Whereas these tracts descend ipsilaterally, they terminate on interneurons whose axons decussate in the ventral commissure and thus influence axial musculature bilaterally.

[2]Most of the projection to the cranial nerve motor nuclei are bilateral; those to the part of the facial nucleus that innervates upper facial muscles are bilateral, and those to the lower facial muscles are contralateral (see Chap. 11).

SOURCE: Martin JH. *Neuroanatomy Text and Atlas.* The McGraw Hill Companies; 2003.

AUDITORY SYSTEM

Sound produces vibrations on the tympanic membrane, which are transmitted to the cochlea via the ossicles (malleus, incus, stapes) (see Fig. 2-25). Signals from the hair cells of the cochlea are transmitted to the cochlear division of cranial nerve VIII. This projects to the superior olivary complex, which transmits to the inferior colliculus by the lateral lemniscus. The medial geniculate nucleus is the thalamic relay nucleus for sound. The primary auditory cortex located on the superior surface of the temporal lobe is known as Heschl's gyrus. Sounds from each ear are processed bilaterally.

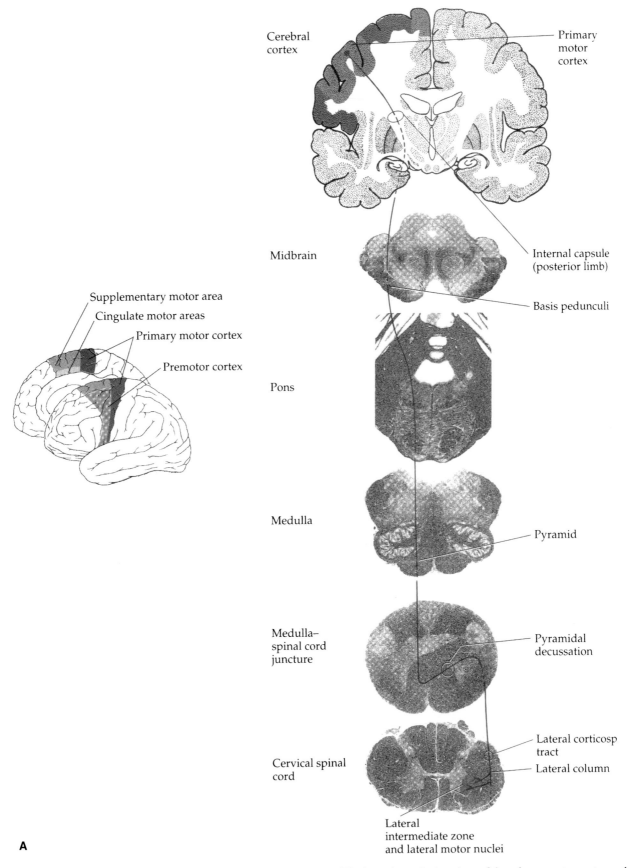

Cerebral cortex

Primary motor cortex

Supplementary motor area

Cingulate motor areas

Primary motor cortex

Premotor cortex

Midbrain

Internal capsule (posterior limb)

Basis pedunculi

Pons

Medulla

Pyramid

Medulla–spinal cord juncture

Pyramidal decussation

Lateral corticosp tract

Lateral column

Cervical spinal cord

Lateral intermediate zone and lateral motor nuclei

A

FIG. 2-24   Laterally descending pathways. **A.** Lateral corticospinal tract. The inset shows the locations of the primary motor cortex and three premotor areas: the supplementary motor area, the cingulate motor areas, and the premotor cortex. **B.** Rubrospinal tract. The lateral corticospinal tract also originates from neurons located in area 6 and the parietal lobe. *(Continued)*

SOURCE: Martin JH. *Neuroanatomy Text and Atlas*. The McGraw Hill Companies; 2003.

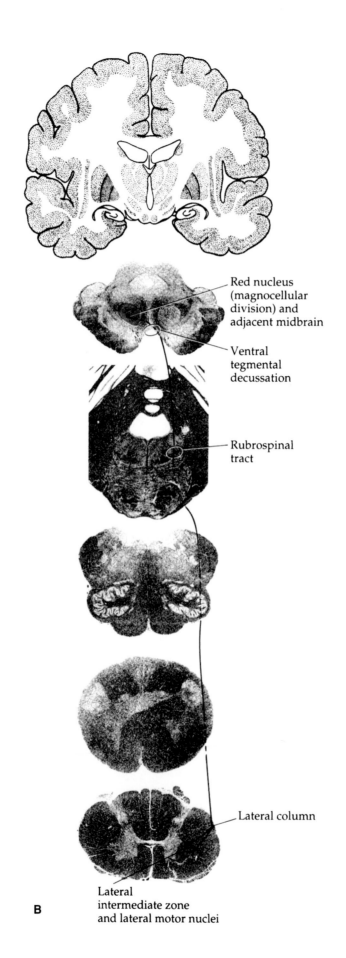

Red nucleus
(magnocellular
division) and
adjacent midbrain

Ventral
tegmental
decussation

Rubrospinal
tract

Lateral column

Lateral
intermediate zone
and lateral motor nuclei

B

FIG. 2-24   *(Continued).*

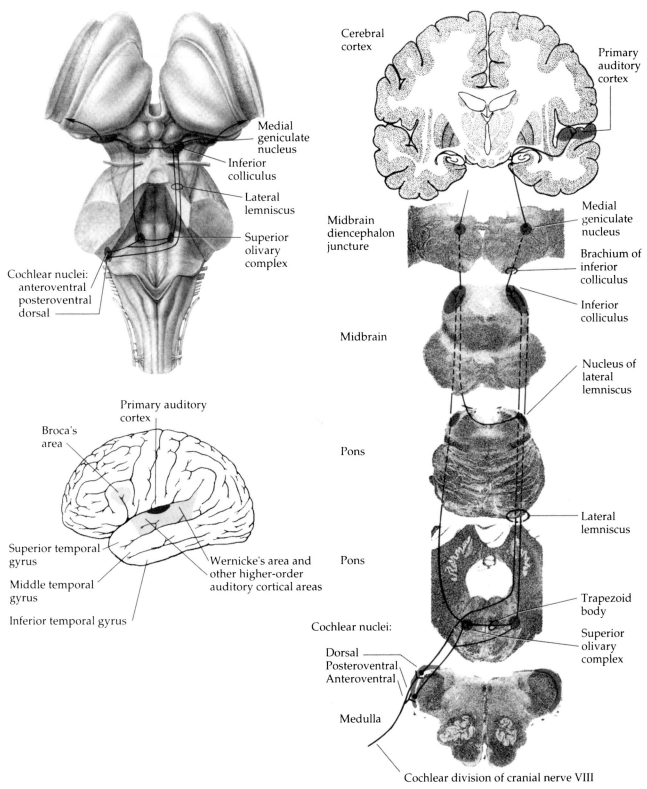

FIG. 2-25 Organization of the auditory system revealed in cross section at different levels through the brain stem and in coronal section through the diencephalon and cerebral hemispheres. The inset shows the auditory and speech-related areas of the cerebral cortex. Wernicke's area, for understanding speech, is located in the superior temporal gyrus. Broca's area, for articulating speech, is located in the inferior frontal gyrus. Heschl's gyri are located within the lateral sulcus and cannot be seen on the surface.
SOURCE: Martin JH. *Neuroanatomy Text and Atlas*. The McGraw Hill Companies; 2003.

REFERENCES

White JS. *USMLE Road Map Neuroscience.* Lange Medical Books/McGraw Hill; 2002.

Martin JH. *Neuroanatomy Text and Atlas.* The McGraw Hill Companies; 2003.

Woolsey TA, Hanaway J, Gado MH. *The Brain Atlas.* Hoboken, NJ: Wiley and Sons; 2003.

Osborne AG. *Diagnostic Cerebral Angiography.* Lippincott Williams and Wilkins;1999.

Lister JR, Rhoton AL Jr, Matsushima T, Peace DA. Microsurgical anatomy of the posterior inferior cerebellar artery, *Neurosurgery.* 1982;10(2):170–99.

Chapter 3

MRI AND CT ARTIFACTS

Understanding common artifacts in computed axial tomography (CT) and magnetic resonance imaging (MRI) is important to properly interpret imaging studies. Common MRI artifacts include aliasing, Gibbs truncation artifact, motion ghosts, susceptibility artifact, and chemical shift artifact.

Aliasing artifact can occur in either the frequency or phase direction. Aliasing in the phase direction occurs when the object being imaged in the phase direction is larger than the field of view. Parts of the object outside the field of view will acquire a phase, which will cause the object to appear on the opposite side of the image (see Fig. 3-1). This artifact can be eliminated by increasing the field of view (called no phase wrap on some scanners) or swapping the phase and frequency directions.

Aliasing in the frequency direction can occur from a failure to sample the MRI signal at twice the highest frequency of the MRI signal. This is not usually a problem on modern MRI scanners.

Gibbs truncation artifact occurs at high contrast interfaces such as the cord/cerebrospinal fluid (CSF) junction. This occurs mathematically from truncation of the sampled MRI signal during Fourier transformation, usually in the phase encoding direction. This artifact can be eliminated by increasing the sampling time, increasing the matrix size in the phase encode direction (increasing the number of phase encoding steps), or decreasing the field of view (and thus decreasing the pixel size). This artifact is most commonly seen in the cervical spine on T2 weighted images (see Fig. 3-2).

Ghosting is an artifact caused by motion (periodic or non-periodic). Examples include pulsation artifact from blood vessels, motion ghosts from respiration, or nonperiodic motions such as eye blinking (see Fig. 3-3). Motion ghosts can be eliminated in a variety of ways, which include cardiac or respiratory gating, flow compensation pulses, and the use of spatial presaturation pulses.

Susceptibility artifact is caused by the presence of magnetic materials that can cause signal loss. Susceptibility artifact arises from distortions in the local magnetic environment, with resultant signal loss and signal distortion (Fig. 3-4). Magnetic susceptibility artifact is less pronounced in spin echo sequences (see Fig. 3-4A) than in gradient echo and echo planar imaging sequences (see Fig. 3-4B).

Chemical shift artifact is caused by the differences in precessional frequency between protons in fat and water molecules and is seen in the frequency encoding direction. Anywhere that fat-containing structures are adjacent to water-containing structures, there can be some misregistration of fat and water molecules, depending on the acquisition parameters (matrix size and band width). This will result in a bright band on the end of the lower frequencies from overlap of fat and water, and a dark band in the region of the higher frequencies.

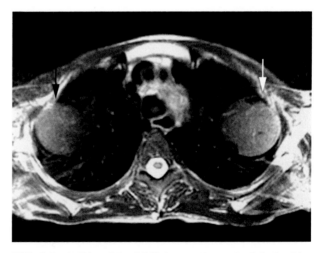

FIG. 3-1 A T1 weighted MR image shows the left shoulder (black arrow) wrapped around to the right side of the chest and the right shoulder (white arrow) wrapped around to the left side of the image.

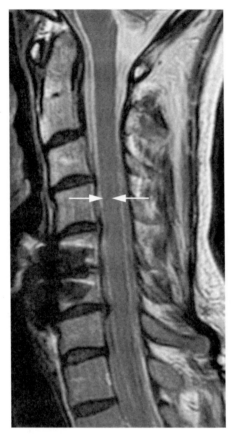

FIG. 3-2 A sagittal T2 weighted image of the cervical spine shows the classic artifactual high signal lines from truncation artifact (white arrows).

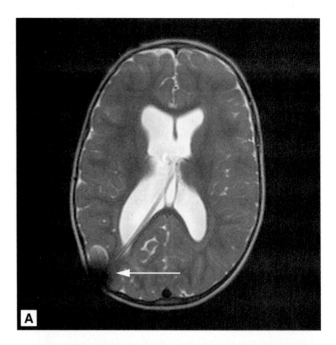

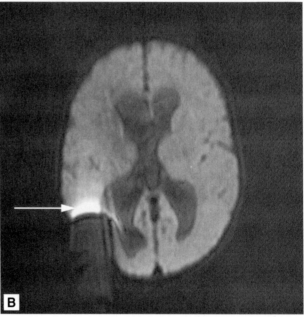

FIG. 3-4 **A.** There is an area of signal loss in the right parietal region at the site of insertion of a ventriculostomy catheter on axial T2 weighted images (white arrow). **B.** The signal loss from susceptibility artifact is more pronounced on echo-planar images (white arrow).

CT ARTIFACTS

A number of artifacts can limit CT scanning. These include artifacts from the image acquisition and processing stages of the examination as well as from patient movement or the presence of a metallic foreign body.

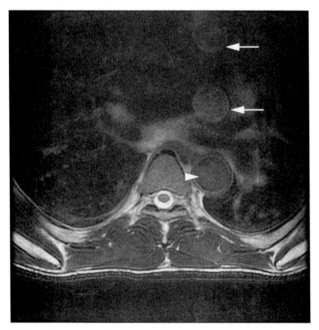

FIG. 3-3 An axial T2 weighted image of the thoracic spine shows motion ghosts (white arrows) from pulsatile flow in the aorta (white arrowhead).

Beam hardening or streak artifact, is characterized by dark bands that appears between dense objects in an image. When photons pass through a dense object, the lower energy photons are preferentially absorbed, leaving only higher energy photons. This is known as beam hardening. The calculated attenuation in a CT detector is the average attenuation of photons of all energies. Reconstructed images therefore show dark lines or streaks between dense objects (see Fig. 3-5). This type of artifact is especially prevalent in the presence of a metallic foreign body, and can be seen with contrast administration as well.

Partial volume artifacts occur at the edge of dense structures, such as bone in the skull base. The resulting artifacts are streak shaped artifacts that are similar in appearance to beam hardening artifacts. They can be reduced by scanning with a lower slice thickness, as is commonly done in the posterior fossa.

Ring artifacts are the creation of a circular artifact from a detector being out of calibration. This artifact has the appearance of concentric rings.

Patient motion can result in streaking of the images. Faster scanning techniques, conscious sedation, and devices that prevent involuntary motion (such as head holders) are usually sufficient to reduce this artifact. Often repeat scanning of images degraded by patient motion is necessary (see Fig. 3-6). Fast scanning speeds (faster gantry rotation, multidetector scanners) also help reduce motion artifacts.

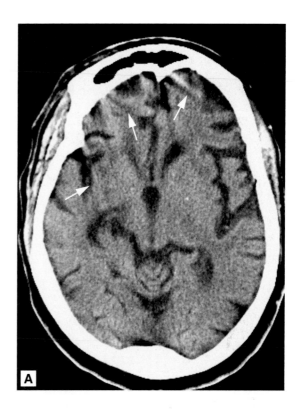

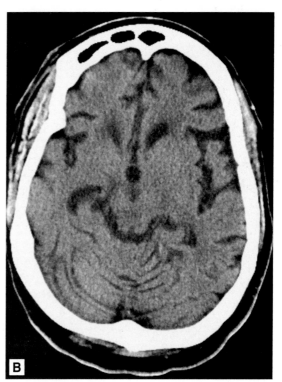

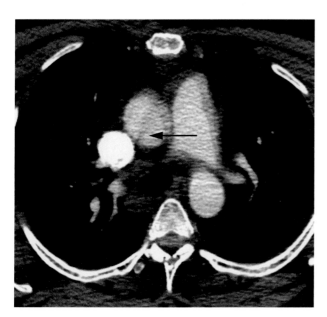

FIG. 3-5 There is an area of "streak artifact" (black arrow) adjacent to the superior vena cava after administration of intravenous contrast. A similar artifact can be seen from partial volume effects at the skull base or from metallic objects.

FIG. 3-6 Patient motion can result in misregistration of the filtered back-projection. **A.** CT image, resulting in dark streaks, similar to those seen in beam hardening artifact (white arrows). **B.** This streak artifact is not present on repeat scanning.

REFERENCES

Liney G. *MRI in Clinical Practice.* London: Springer-Verlag; 2006.

Hashemi RH, Bradley WG. *MRI: The Basics.* Baltimore, MD: Williams and Wilkens; 1997.

Barrett JF, Keat N. Artifacts in CT: Recognition and Avoidance. *Radiographics.* 2004; 24(6):1679–91.

Raupach R, Flohr T. Artifacts in Multislice CT. In *Protocols for Multislice CT.* Bruening R, Kuettner A, Flohr T eds. Berlin: Springer-Verlag 2006.

Chapter 4

STROKE

CASE 4-1

A 75-year-old woman had been admitted to the hospital by her family practice physician for transient blurry vision in the right eye. A head CT performed on admission was significant for a small right frontal hypodensity thought to represent a subacute or chronic stroke (see Figs. 4-1-1–4-1-5). The next day the patient abruptly developed a headache, accompanied by a severe left-sided hemiparesis, and neglect. A repeat head CT was performed and the patient was treated with tissue plasminogen activator (tPA). She failed to show any improvement in response to the treatment.

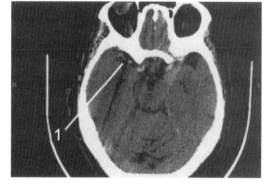

FIG. 4-1-2 Head CT performed at the time of left hemiparesis onset. The study is significant for a hyperdense right middle cerebral artery (1) suggesting that it contains clot.

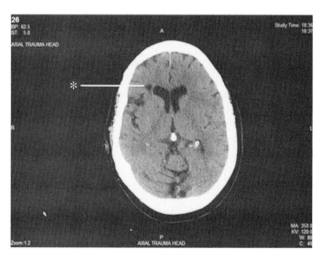

FIG. 4-1-1 Original head CT performed on admission suggesting the presence of a subacute or chronic right frontal lacunar stroke (*).

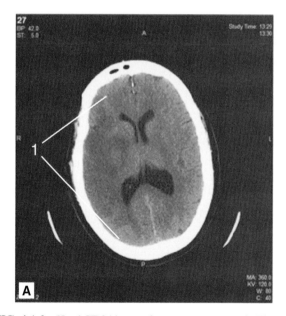

FIG. 4-1-3 Head CT 24 hours after symptom onset. **A.** There is a diffuse hypodensity involving portions of the frontal, temporal and parietal lobes (1).

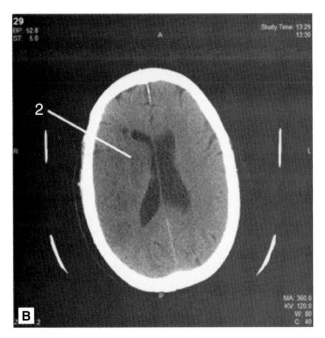

FIG. 4-1-3 B. Some mass effect (2) is seen, indicating edema.

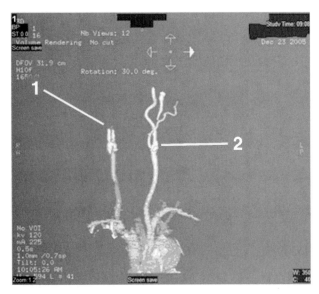

FIG. 4-1-4 CT angiography clearly demonstrating a large calcified plaque and complete occlusion of the right internal and external carotid arteries (1) just distal to the bifurcation. Some calcification is also apparent at the left carotid bulb (2).

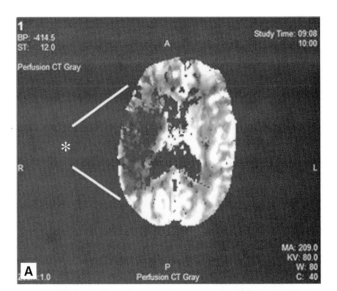

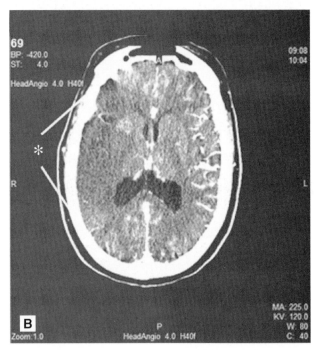

FIG. 4-1-5 A. CT angiography and perfusion study revealed low blood flow in the distribution of the middle cerebral artery (*). **B.** The anterior cerebral artery territory is preserved through the anterior communicating artery serving as a passage for blood flow from the contralateral side.

Clinical-Radiological Diagnosis: Right internal carotid occlusion and middle cerebral artery distribution stroke.

KEY FACTS

Head CT may not show brain parenchyma changes following acute stroke. CT perfusion/angiography may be useful.

CASE 4-2

A 68-year-old woman with a history of hypertension and atrial fibrillation presents to the emergency room with left body weakness, decreased level of consciousness, and slurred speech. The onset was sudden, approximately 4 hours ago, while eating dinner with her husband. Examination findings include blood pressure of 200/95, dysarthria, corticospinal pattern of left body weakness (face and upper extremity worse than lower extremity), and left side neglect.

Neuroimaging is shown in Figs. 4-2-1–4-2-3

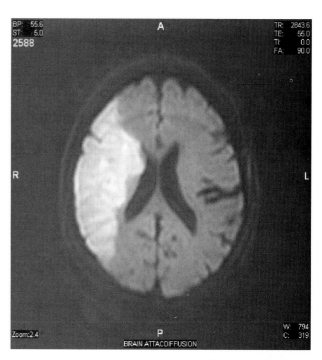

FIG. 4-2-2 Diffusion weighted MRI. High signal is clearly demonstrated in the right MCA territory.

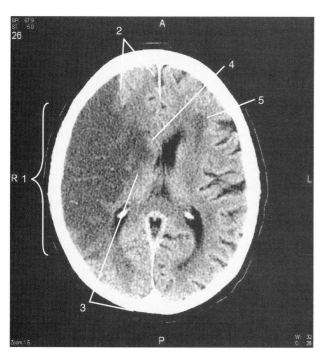

FIG. 4-2-1 Noncontrast head CT. There is a hypodensity in the distribution (1) of the right middle cerebral artery (MCA) territory. Notice the sparing of the areas of brain perfused by the anterior (2) and posterior (3) cerebral arteries. It is common for such a large infarct to be accompanied by brain edema. In this case the right lateral ventricle is compressed by a mild amount of brain swelling (4). This swelling will generally increase over the next 2–3 days. A small hypodensity seen in the left hemisphere (5) most likely is due to a subacute or chronic infarct unrelated to the present clinical presentation.

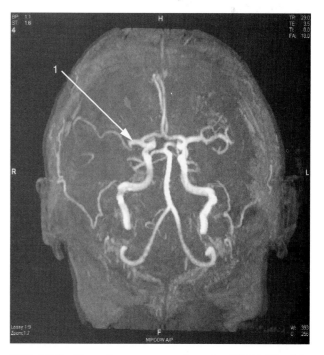

FIG. 4-2-3 Magnetic resonance angiography (MRA). The right MCA can be seen ending abruptly just before its bifurcation (1). This is the point where occlusion occurred, most likely due to an embolus. All of the other major intracranial blood vessels can be seen intact.

Clinical-Radiological Diagnosis: Right middle cerebral artery stroke.

KEY FACTS

The typical CT finding within several to 24 hours of an acute stroke is hypodensity in the area of infarction. Diffusion weighted MRI is the most sensitive neuroimaging test available for assisting with the diagnosis of acute stroke.

CASE 4-3

A 56-year-old man had begun to feel "drunk" while driving his car. Once he arrived home he noticed the feeling of "pins-and-needles" in his left upper extremity. Over the course of several hours the symptoms evolved to the point where he had slurred speech, and weakness of his left upper and lower extremities. Examination findings included a mild upper motor neuron pattern of weakness involving the left body, dysarthria, and left body sensory loss.

Neuroimaging is shown in Figs. 4-3-1 to 4-3-3

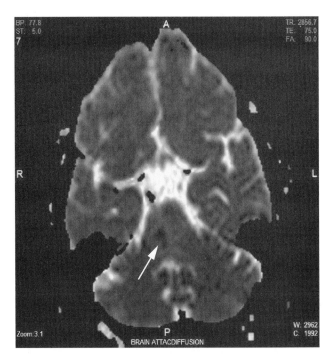

FIG. 4-3-2 Apparent diffusion coefficient (ADC) MRI demonstrates a corresponding area of low signal. This confirms the acute cellular damage, supporting the diagnosis of stroke in this case.

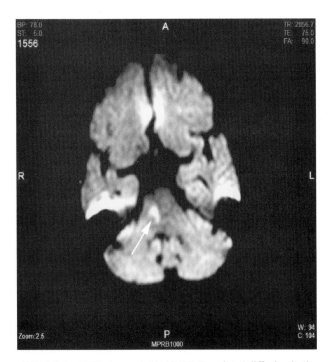

FIG. 4-3-1 Diffusion weighted MRI. Restricted diffusion in the right pons is indicated by abnormal signal.

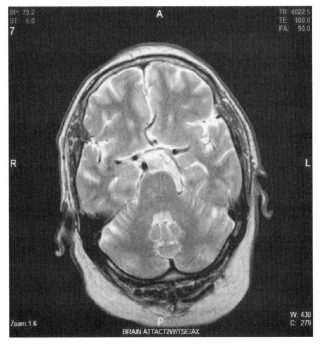

FIG. 4-3-3 T2 TSE MRI. Very mild high signal in the right pons. This is also confirmatory that the right pontine lesion is acute.

Clinical-Radiological Diagnosis: Motor sensory stroke due to right pontine infarct.

KEY FACTS

Restricted diffusion with normal T2 signal is the hallmark of acute stroke.

CASE 4-4

An 86-year-old woman is brought in to the emergency room because of a "new" right-sided weakness. The nursing home staff had noticed over the past day that she was not moving the right side of her body as well as usual. She has had some sort of difficulty with speech for at least the past 2 years. Examination is significant for a nonfluent aphasia with relatively preserved repetition and a mild right body upper motor neuron pattern of hemiparesis involving the face, arm, and leg. Significant laboratory findings included a large amount of white blood cells and bacteria in her urine.

Neuroimaging is shown in Figs. 4-4-1–4-4-2

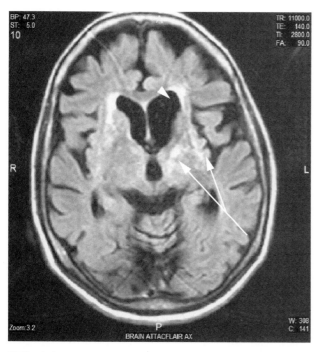

FIG. 4-4-1 Fluid attenuation inversion recovery (FLAIR) sequence MRI demonstrating abnormal high signal in the periventricular white matter and left basal ganglia/internal capsule/thalamus (arrows). The deep nuclei and internal capsule lesions are in an anatomical location which may explain her symptoms and most likely indicate infarcts in this clinical setting. The age of the infarcts are difficult to determine with certainty, however they are at least several hours. The dilatation of the left lateral ventricle (arrowhead) is most likely ex vacuo suggesting that the infarcts are chronic.

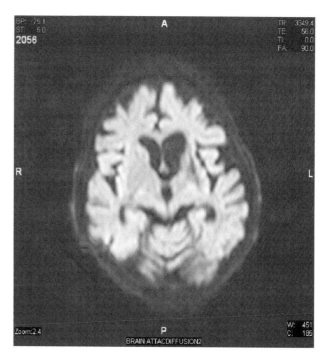

FIG. 4-4-2 Diffusion-weighted image (DWI) fails to show any areas of abnormal high signal indicating that the lesions are not new. Additionally, there is an area of low signal in the left putamen, also consistent with a chronic infarct.

Clinical-Radiological Diagnosis: Reemergence of symptoms related to an old stroke in the setting of an infection (urinary tract in this case).

KEY FACTS

Chronic strokes may have high T2 signal without restricted diffusion.

CASE 4-5

A 48-year-old-diabetic man is found down, covered in emesis. He was profoundly hypoxic on admission to the emergency room where he was intubated. His blood sugar was extremely low. On admission the patient had a Glasgow coma scale of 3. He remained comatose throughout his hospitalization, and had diffuse slowing on EEG.

Neuroimaging is shown in Figs 4-5-1–4-5-3

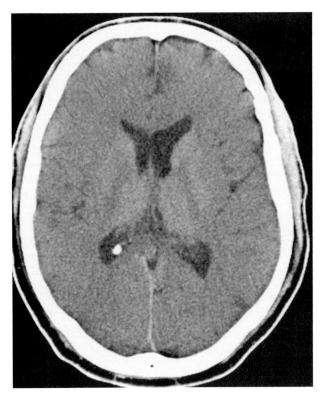

FIG. 4-5-1 The patient's initial head CT shows diffuse loss of grey/white differentiation in the frontal, parietal, and occipital lobes, sparing the thalami bilaterally as well as both caudate lobes and internal capsules.

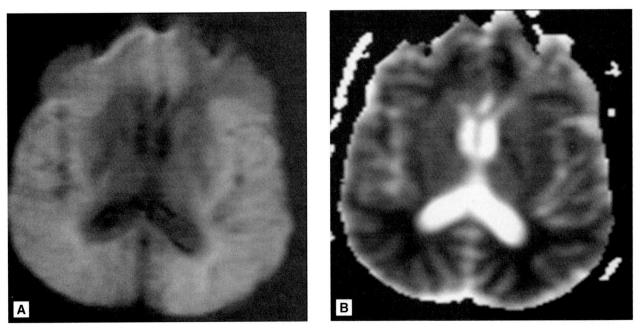

FIG. 4-5-2 **A.** Diffusion weighted images using non-standard windows (as sent to the picture archiving and communication system (PACS) by the MRI technologist) demonstrate relatively increased signal within the cerebral cortex and the underlying subcortical white matter diffusely, sparing a portion of the left frontal lobe, the internal capsules, and the caudate heads bilaterally. **B.** The apparent diffusion coefficient (ADC) map shows diffuse restricted diffusion with sparing of a portion the left frontal lobe, the internal capsules, and the caudate heads.

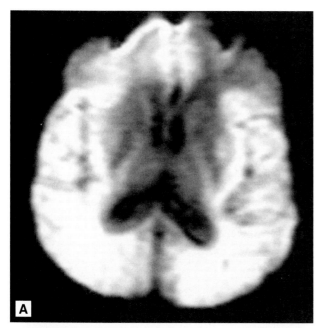

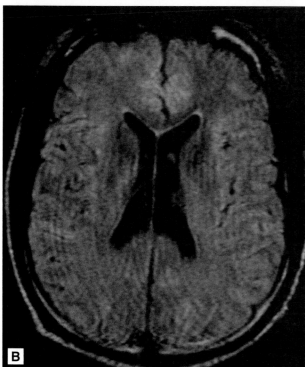

FIG. 4-5-3 **A.** The diffusion weighted images, when windowed the standard window width and level (Width 250, Level 150) shows marked gross signal abnormality. **B.** FLAIR images show increased signal within the gray matter bilaterally in the frontal, parietal, and occipital regions.

Clinical-Radiological Diagnosis: Diffuse Hypoxic Ischemic Encephalopathy.

KEY FACTS

Diffuse anoxic brain injury can occur secondary to cardiac arrest, respiratory failure, strangulation, drowning,

or other causes of a global ischemic insult. T1, T2, and FLAIR images may show abnormal signal within the cortical grey matter and subcortical white matter.

Diffusion weighted imaging is a very sensitive way to detect early ischemic changes. However, improperly windowed diffusion images can have a deceptively unremarkable appearance. Often the windows on diffusion images will be adjusted to a normal appearance rather than to a standard window width and level (Window Width/Level: 250/150 at our institution). Because the diffusion signal abnormality is symmetric, this can artificially make this a more difficult radiological diagnosis.

REFERENCE

McKinney AM, Teksam M, Felice R, et al. Diffusion Weighted Imaging in the Setting of Diffuse Cortical Laminar Necrosis and Hypoxic Ischemic Encephalopathy. *AJNR. Am J Neuroradiol.* 2004;196–1665.

CASE 4-6

A 36-year-old right-handed woman presented in November 2000 with multiple episodes of nonfluent aphasia with right arm heaviness. The patient was admitted to the hospital and found to have a left cerebral infarct and left MCA stenosis. The patient was started on clopidogrel. She then had a recurrent left MCA TIA despite compliance with medical therapy.

Neuroimaging is shown in Figs. 4-6-1–4-6-3

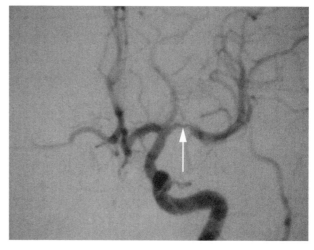

FIG. 4-6-1 There is a high grade stenosis (65%) of the M1 segment of the left middle cerebral artery (arrow).

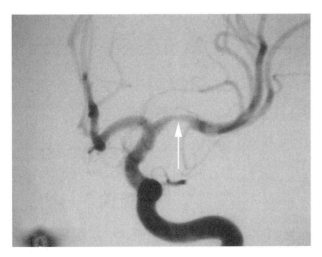

FIG. 4-6-2 Postangioplasty there is improvement in vessel caliber.

Clinical-Radiological Diagnosis: Intracranial atherosclerotic disease.

KEY FACTS

Optimal medical management of patients with intracranial atherosclerotic disease has been the subject of a long-standing debate in the neurologic community. Advances in endovascular technology have made intracranial angioplasty and stenting for atherosclerotic stenoses technically feasible. Preliminary data on intracranial angioplasty and stenting have shown these procedures to be associated with high rates of in-stent re-stenosis. Despite this problem, intracranial angioplasty

and stenting have been advocated as therapeutic options for symptomatic patients who have failed medical therapy as well as for some asymptomatic patients with high-grade intracranial atherosclerotic stenoses because of the poor prognosis for initial and recurrent stroke while on medical therapy alone.

Case courtesy of DeWitte T. Cross, MD

REFERENCES

Chimovitz M, Lynn M, Howlett Smith H, et al. Comparison of warfarin and aspirin for symptomatic intracranial arterial stenosis. *NEJM.* 2005;352:1305–16.

Gomez C, Orr S. Angioplasty and stenting for primary treatment of intracranial arterial stenoses. *Arch Neurol.* 2001; 58:1687–90.

Lutsep H, Barnwell S, Mawad M. Stenting of symptomatic atherosclerotic lesion in the vertebral or intracranial arteries (SSYLVIA): study results. *Stroke.* 2004;35(6):138–1392.

Thijs V, Albers G. Symptomatic Intracranial stenosis outcome of patients who fail antithrombotic therapy. *Neurology.* 2000; 55:490–97.

Wityk R, Lehman D, Klag M, et al. Race and Sex Differences in the Distribution of Cerebral Atherosclerosis. *Stroke.* 1996;197–1980.

CASE 4-7

The patient is a 62-year-old man who was found to have decreased awareness, difficulty with speech, and right-sided arm and leg weakness 4 hours prior to arrival in the emergency room. The patient had a National Institute of Health Stroke Scale score of 20 on arrival to the emergency room. The patient had a known old left occipital stroke. The admission head CT was otherwise unremarkable.

Neuroimaging is shown in Figs. 4-7-1 to 4-7-3

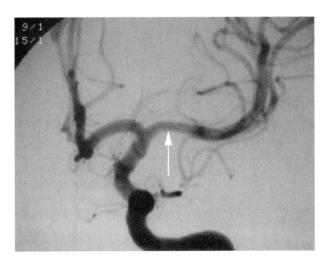

FIG. 4-6-3 After placement of a 2.5 mm × 10 mm stent, there is no evidence of residual stenosis (white arrow).

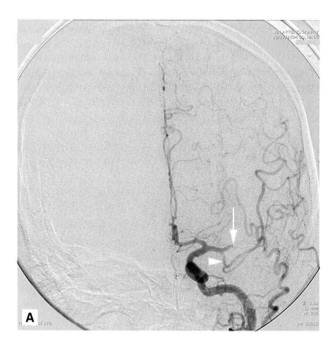

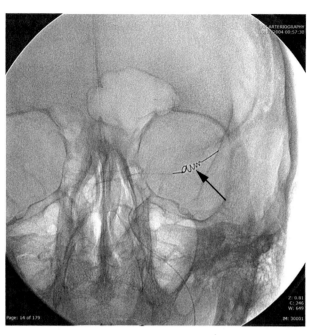

FIG. 4-7-2 A spot image shows the snare-like MERCI retriever device (black arrow) advanced into the clot in the left middle cerebral artery.

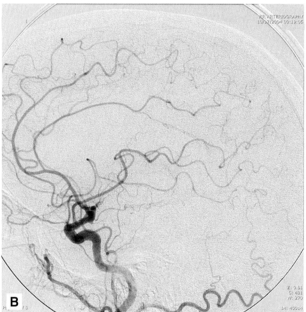

FIG. 4-7-1 **A.** A conventional angiogram with AP and **B.** Lateral images from a left common carotid artery injection shows occlusion of the left middle cerebral artery (white arrow) beyond the origin of the anterior temporal artery (arrowhead). Note the absence of filling of the middle cerebral artery on the lateral angiogram (B).

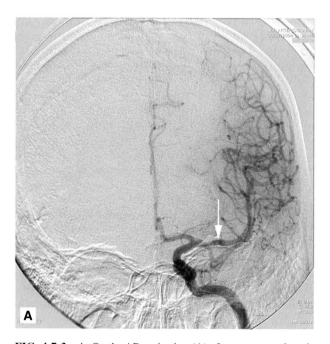

FIG. 4-7-3 **A.** On the AP projection (A) after treatment there is normal filling of the left MCA (white arrow), as well as **B.** The distal branches (black arrows) seen best on the lateral projection. The patient made a complete neurologic recovery.

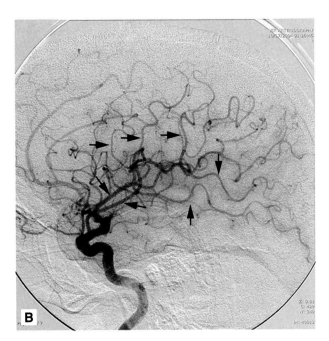

FIG. 4-7-3 (*Continued*)

Clinical-Radiological Diagnosis: Left middle cerebral artery occlusion treated by endovascular means.

KEY FACTS

The current standard of care for ischemic stroke patients is intravenous thrombolytic administration within 3 hours of stroke onset. However this limited time frame only allows a small number of patients to be treated. In large vessel occlusions, the overall outcomes without treatment is extremely poor. It is known that areas of salvageable brain tissue are present beyond the currently accepted 3-hour treatment window. There is some data suggesting that intra-arterial thrombolytics may allow the therapeutic window to be extended to 6 hours. Some novel endovascular devices such as the MERCI retriever device appear to be a promising approach.

Case courtesy of Ronald Budzik.

REFERENCES

NINDS rt-PA Stroke Group. Tissue plasminogen activator for acute ischemic stroke. *NEJM*. 1995;333:1581–87.

del Zoppo GJ, Higashida RT, Furlan AJ, et al. PROACT: a phase ii randomized trial of recombinant pro-urokinase by direct arterial delivery in acute middle cerebral artery stroke. *Stroke* 1998; 29:4–11.

Smith WS, Sung G, Starkman S, et al. Safety and efficacy of mechanical embolectomy in acute ischemic stroke: results of the MERCI trial. *Stroke*. 2005 Jul;36(7):1432–8.

Chapter 5

TUMORS

CASE 5-1

A 34-year-old woman presents with the subacute onset of an occipital headache. The pain is moderate but does not improve with common analgesic drugs and does not spontaneously resolve over 6 weeks. Past medical history is remarkable for subtotal thyroidectomy performed 2 years ago due to thyroid adenocarcinoma. Surgery was followed by local radiation therapy and chemotherapy. Metastatic survey 6 months before the onset of headache failed to show evidence of metastatic disease.

Neuroimaging is shown in Fig. 5-1-1

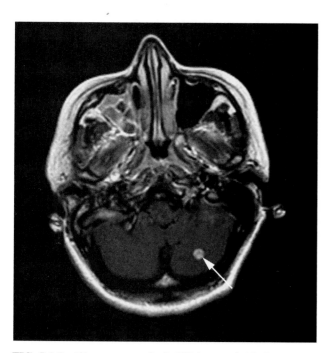

FIG. 5-1-1 T1 postcontrast brain MR is remarkable for a small, round, contrast-enhancing lesion in the left cerebellar hemisphere.

Clinical-Radiological Diagnosis: Metastatic lesion.

KEY FACTS

A medical history of recent malignancy combined with an isolated, round, enhancing brain lesion is highly suggestive of metastasis.

The imaging characteristics of metastatic lesion include ring-enhancing lesions, commonly found at the gray-white matter interface. The most common infratentorial neoplasm in adults is a metastatic lesion. However, metastatic lesions are more commonly supratentorial. Though the presence of multiple lesions favors metastases versus a primary brain tumor, nearly half of supratentorial metastatic lesions will present as a solitary lesion. Metastatic lesions can present as calcified, hemorrhagic, or dural-based lesions.

CASE 5-2

A 54-year-old man reports the sudden onset of double vision. Neurological examination reveals ptosis and inability to look inward in the right eye associated with inability to look outward of the left eye. The visual fields show a pattern of concentric restriction on the right eye (in association with reduction of visual acuity) combined with upper hemianopsia on the left eye. These findings suggest the presence of a lesion affecting the optic (II) and oculomotor (III) nerves on the right side, the abducens (VI) on the left side, and the optic chiasm.

Neuroimaging is shown in Figs. 5-2-1–5-2-2.

Clinical-Radiological Diagnosis: Meningioma of the clivus.

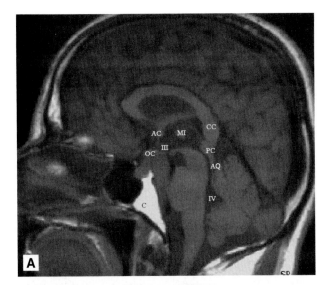

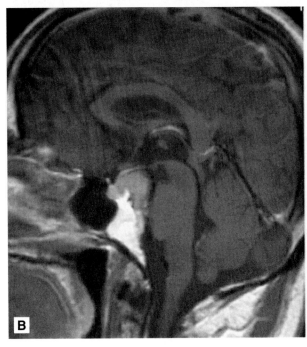

FIG. 5-2-1 **A.** Precontrast and **B.** post-contrast sagittal T1 MRI. These images are taken on the midline (as shown by many landmarks: the anterior (AC) and posterior commissure (PC), the thalamic massa intermedia (MI), the corpus callosum (CC), the aqueduct of Sylvius (AQ), the third (III) and fourth (IV) ventricles). An homogeneous contrast enhancing lesion originating from the upper clivus (C) and growing upward toward the optic chiasm (OC) is readily detected.

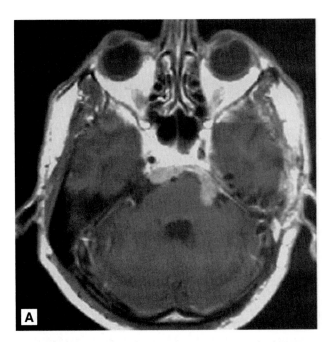

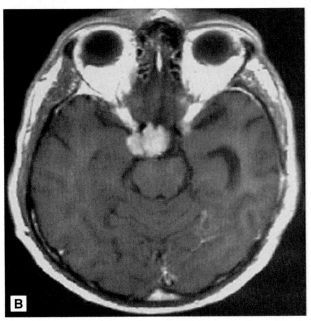

FIG. 5-2-2 Axial postcontrast T1: The lesion originates from the clivus indenting the pons on the left side but also grows upward toward the right optic nerve. This complex growth pattern explains the involvement of the 6th nerve on the left and of the 3rd nerve on the right side.

KEY FACTS

Although slow growing meningiomas may present acutely. They are commonly dural and enhance uniformly. Common imaging features of meningiomas are high attenuation on CT, sometimes with calcification, homogenous enhancement after contrast administration, the presence of a dural tail, and adjacent bony hyperostosis. On MRI imaging they tend to be hypointense on T1-weighted images, enhance homogenously, be slightly hyperintense on T2-weighted images, and have a dural tail on post contrast images. A differential for a mass lesion originating from the clivus includes chordoma, chondrosarcoma, metastasis, or plasmacytoma.

CASE 5-3

A 41-year-old man presents with headaches.
Neuroimaging is shown in Figs. 5-3-1–5-3-3.

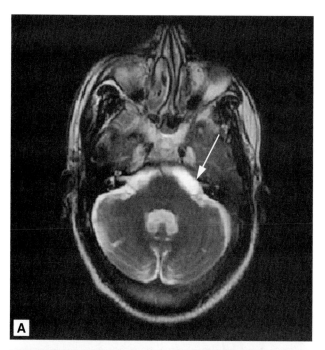

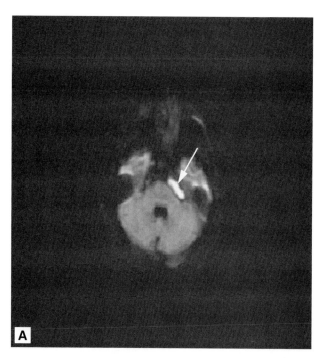

FIG. 5-3-2   A. Diffusion weighted images show bright signal (white arrow) in the left prepontine cistern.

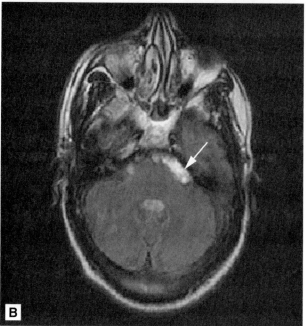

FIG. 5-3-1   A. Axial T2 weighted images show a high signal intensity lesion in the left prepontine cistern (white arrow) compared to the CSF. **B.** The lesion is also high signal intensity on FLAIR (fluid attenuation inversion recovery) images (white arrow), while CSF is dark.

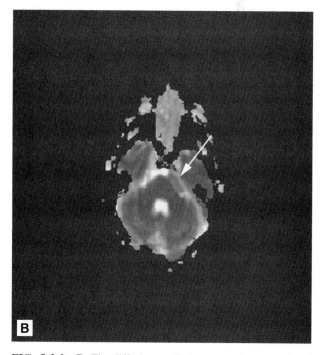

FIG. 5-3-2   B. The diffusion coefficient map shows restricted diffusion in the left prepontine cistern mass (white arrow).

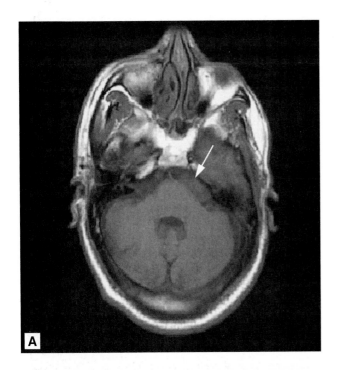

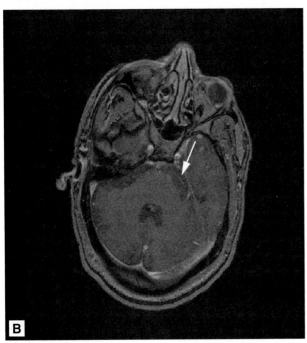

FIG. 5-3-3 On **A.** precontrast images **B.** postcontrast T1 weighted images there is no enhancement in the left prepontine cistern mass (white arrow).

Clinical-Radiological Diagnosis: Epidermoid tumor.

KEY FACTS

The primary differential in this case of a cystic extra-axial mass lesion in the prepontine cistern is an arachnoid cyst or an epidermoid cyst. Epidermoid tumors, like arachnoid cysts are benign lesions. They tend to insinuate themselves between blood vessels and nerves. Epidermoid tumors usually will be hyperintense to the normal cerebrospinal fluid on T1 and T2 weighted images, as opposed to arachnoid cysts, which will follow the cerebrospinal fluid on all sequences. However epidermoid tumors can most easily be distinguished from arachnoid cysts on FLAIR images or diffusion weighted images. Epidermoid cysts will have restricted diffusion on diffusion-weighted imaging and will have high signal on FLAIR images.

REFERENCE

Tsuruda JS, Chew WM, Moseley ME, et al. Diffusion weighted MR imaging of the brain: value of differentiating between extra-axial cysts and epidermoid tumors. *Am J Rosentgenol.* 1990;155:1059–65.

CASE 5-4

A 54-year-old woman undergoes resection of an enlarging nevus on the left shoulder. Pathology reveals a malignant melanoma. After 1 year, she suddenly develops headache, nausea, and vomiting associated with midriasis of the right pupil and fast deterioration of mental state. She is brought to the emergency room of a local hospital and a noncontrast head CT reveals a large hyperdense lesion extending over the pole of the left frontal lobe. A craniotomy is immediately arranged and the lesion, originally thought to be an intraparenchymal haematoma, is removed. Operative findings are remarkable for the presence of a haemorragic core surrounded by a ring of necrosis, with extensive lobar edema. The patient wakes up without focal neurological deficits. At this point, a contrast head CT is obtained, followed by a brain MRI.

Neuroimaging is shown in Figs. 5-4-1–5-4-3.

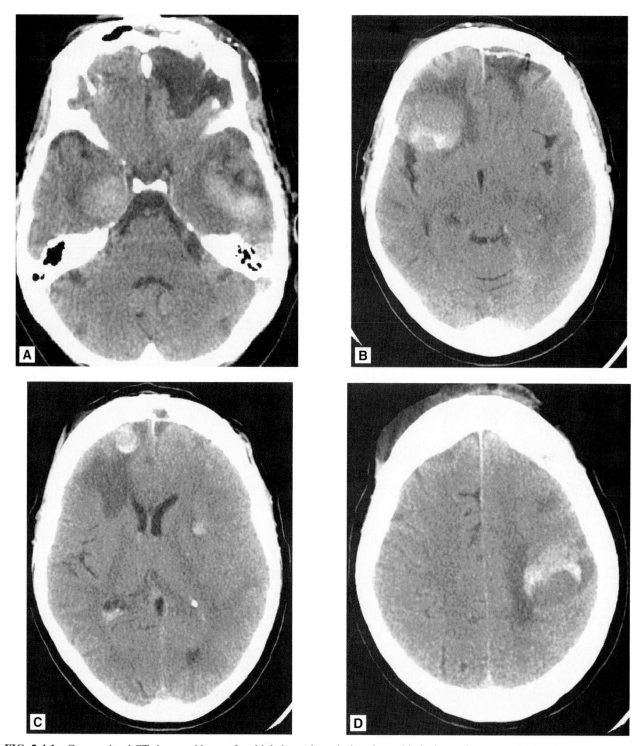

FIG. 5-4-1   Contrast head CT shows evidence of multiple hyperdense lesions located in both anterior temporal lobes **A.** the anterior and inferior aspect of the right frontal lobe **B.** right polar frontal lobe, right parieto-occipital junction at the atrium of the lateral ventricle and left frontal lobe adjacent to the outer margin of the putamen **C.** posterior left frontal lobe **D.** The resection cavity from the left frontal lobe is present in A and B. The lesions display a variety of shapes, homogeneity, and contrast enhancement. The largest lesions are surrounded by a variably wide area of hypodensity suggestive of vasogenic edema (see the right orbito-frontal lesion in B). However, smaller lesions can be surrounded by edema as well (see the right frontopolar lesion in C).

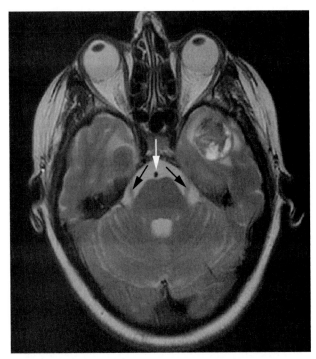

FIG. 5-4-2 Axial T2 MR taken at the level of the trigeminal nerves (black arrows). The basilar artery can be appreciated as a round structure just anterior to the pons (white arrow). Bilateral rounded lesions in the temporal lobes can be appreciated. The right temporal lesion has hypointense signal on T2 weighted images, while the left lesion in the anterior most part of the temporal pole is characterized by marked heterogenous signal, with dark and bright areas suggestive of blood products of different ages. Both lesions are surrounded by a rim of vasogenic edema, characterized as high T2 signal.

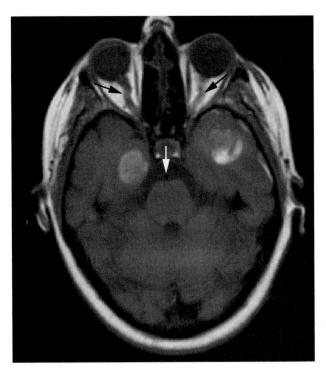

FIG. 5-4-3 Axial T1 precontrast MRI: this cut is slightly higher compared to the axial T2 MRI previously shown: the trigeminal nerves are not visible anymore; both optic nerves can be seen (black arrows). The basilar artery is visible as a signal void, the vessel lumen, surrounded by a ring (white arrow), the vessel wall.

Both of the temporal lesions are hyperintense but the left one is highly heterogenous with hypointense spots and a brighter region posteriorly (suggestive of recent bleeding). Such high signal intensity on T1 weighted images can be seen secondary to blood products or from the presence of melanin in the metastatic lesion.

Clinical-Radiological Diagnosis: Metastatic melanoma.

KEY FACTS

This case is an example of the extremely aggressive course of metastatic melanoma. Multiple brain metastases are very common and invariably fatal due to their poor response to chemo- and radiotherapy. Intralesional necrosis and bleeding associated with poor gadolinium enhancement are quite characteristic of brain metastatic melanoma. Melanoma, renal cell cancer, choriocarcinoma, and thyroid cancer are common hemorrhagic metastatic lesions.

CASE 5-5

A 35-year-old woman has chronic occipital headaches and modest swallowing difficulties with solid food. The pain has a deep, constant character with a steadily worsening observed over the 2 months. Neurological examination is remarkable for trigeminal hypoesthesia. On an occasion of an acute episode of pain, a noncontrast head CT is obtained revealing a lesion located in the posterior fossa.

Neuroimaging is shown in Figs. 5-5-1–5-5-5.

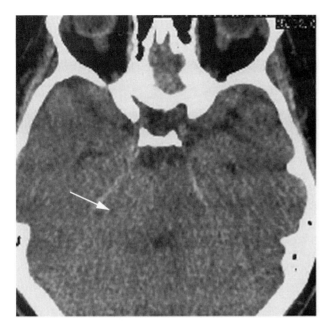

FIG. 5-5-1 Noncontrast head CT. A slightly hyperdense ellipsoidal lesion attached to the posterior surface of the tentorium can be appreciated on the right side arrow. Midbrain is displaced laterally against the opposite tentorial surface and displays low attenuation suggesting the presence of edema related to the compression. The hypodensity partially surrounds the fourth ventricle, which is modestly displaced but remains open. The temporal horns of the lateral ventricles do not appear to be enlarged and the cisternal spaces are open.

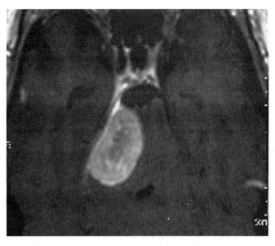

FIG. 5-5-3 Axial post-contrast T1 MRI. The lesion shows avid contrast enhancement. The lesion has a broad based dural attachment, with a dural tail.

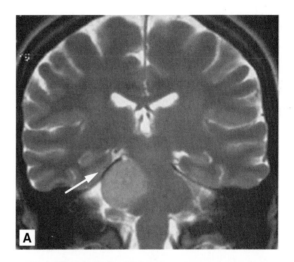

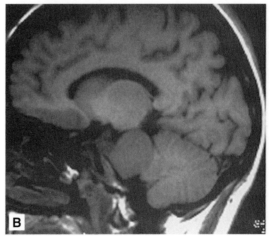

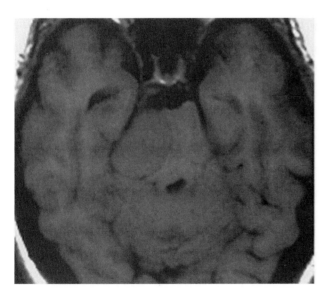

FIG. 5-5-2 Precontrast axial T1 MRI. A homogenous slightly hypointense ellipsoidal mass located between the tentorium and the brainstem. This lesion displaces but does not invade the midbrain. Note the presence of a CSF cleft separating the mass lesion from the brain parenchyma. This is a sign of an extra-axial mass lesion.

FIG. 5-5-4 **A.** Coronal T2 MRI and **B.** Sagittal T1 MRI. The tentorial origin of the lesion can be clearly seen on these image (arrow). On the coronal cut (A), upward displacement of the tentorium can be seen (compare with the opposite side, where the tentorium convexity is directed downward). Both the midbrain and pons are displaced laterally. This lesion has high signal intensity on T2 weighted images, and low signal on T1 weighted images, which is common in meningiomas.

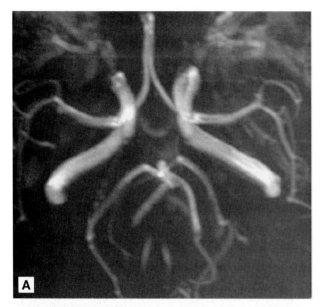

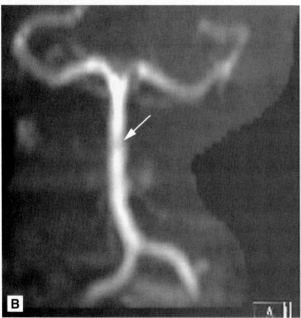

FIG. 5-5-5 A. MRA of the circle of Willis. **B.** Detail of the basilar artery. Despite the large size of this posterior fossa lesion, there is no substantial displacement of the vertebro-basilar complex. The basilar artery (white arrow) has a straight course while the right vertebral artery is slightly pushed to the left. No gross displacement of the supratentorial intracranial vessels can be appreciated.

Clinical-Radiological diagnosis: Tentorial meningioma.

KEY FACTS

Meningiomas are the most common extra-axial tumor. Most are supratentorial. A tentorial lesion can involve both sides of the tentorium. The tentorial base, uniform contrast enhancement, and lack of parenchymal infiltration

all strongly suggested the diagnosis in this case. Meningiomas have a classic angiographic appearance. They may have blood supply from the internal or external carotid artery, depending on their location. On angiography they have a sunburst appearance, with early brisk enhancement, and delayed wash out.

Common imaging features of meningiomas include high density on CT, sometimes with calcification, homogenous enhancement after contrast administration, the presence of a dural tail, and adjacent bony hyperostosis. On MRI, they tend to be hypointense on T1 weighted images, enhance homogenously, be slightly hyperintense on T2 weighted images, and have a dural tail on post contrast images.

CASE 5-6

A 50-year-old woman with a known history of a brain tumor had an MRI performed for follow-up evaluation. Neuroimaging is shown in Figs. 5-6-1–5-6-2.

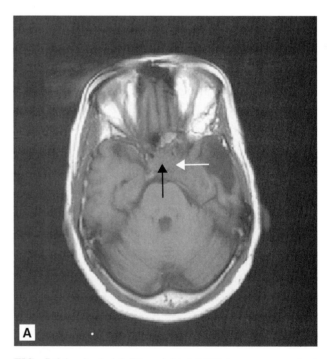

FIG. 5-6-1 A. Axial T1 weighted MRI images precontrast show a hypointense (to white matter) mass lesion in the left cavernous sinus (white arrow), surrounding the left internal carotid artery, and extending across the supra-sellar region (black arrow). **B.** There is homogenous enhancement after contrast administration (white arrow) of the mass lesion in the left cavernous sinus. Note the expansion of the left cavernous sinus. The left internal carotid artery is narrowed. *(Continued)*

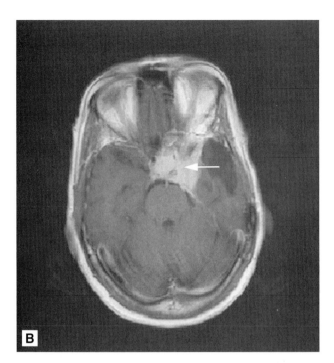

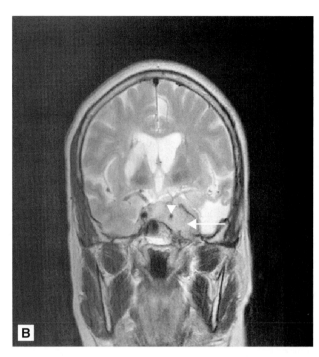

FIG. 5-6-1 *(Continued)*

FIG. 5-6-2 *(Continued)*

Clinical-Radiological Diagnosis: Cavernous sinus meningioma extending into the sella.

KEY FACTS

A meningioma that originates in the cavernous sinus can invade the sella. Meningiomas classically encase and narrow vessels while a pituitary adenoma would not. Cavernous sinus meningiomas that encase and narrow the carotid artery are difficult to resect surgically.

REFERENCE

Hirsch WL, Sekhar LN, Lanzino G, et al. Meningiomas involving the cavernous sinus: value of imaging for predicting surgical complications. *AJR.* 1993;160:1083–88.

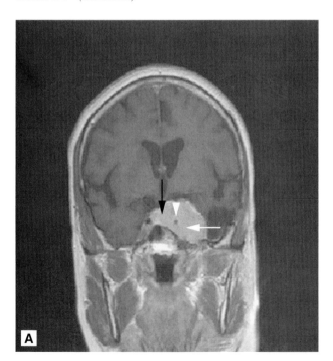

FIG. 5-6-2 A. Postcontrast coronal T1 weighted MRI shows a homogenously enhancing mass in the left cavernous sinus (white arrow) extending across the sella to the right cavernous sinus (black arrow). Note the narrowing of the left internal carotid artery (white arrowhead). **B.** Coronal T2 weighted images also show a left cavernous sinus and sellar mass lesion, hyperintense to gray matter (white arrow) narrowing the left internal carotid artery (white arrowhead). *(Continued)*

CASE 5-7

A 7-year-old child reports the subacute onset of headache, generalized weakness, and psychomotor slowing without focal neurological deficits.

Neuroimaging is shown in Fig. 5-7-1.

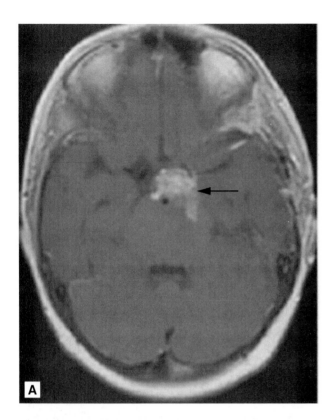

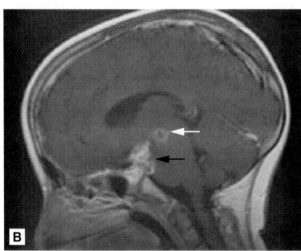

FIG. 5-7-1 **A.** Axial, **B.** Sagittal, and **C.** Coronal T1 MRIs. show a contrast enhancing heterogeneous lesion originanting from the brain/stem with an intra- and extra-axial component. The extra-axial component is characterized by exophytic growth in the chiasmatic cistern (black arrow), predominantly on the left side. The smaller intra-axial component is located at the ponto-mesencephalic junction (white arrow). *(Continued)*

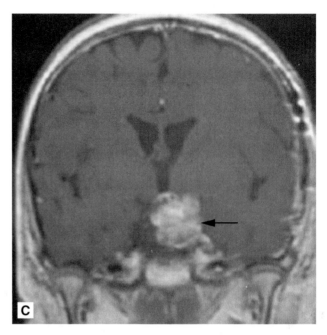

FIG. 5-7-1 *(Continued)*

Clinical-Radiological-Pathological Diagnosis: Low grade glioma. Pathology was performed on a specimen obtained through an open biopsy confirming a WHO grade II glioma.

KEY FACTS

Brainstem gliomas constitute 10–20% of pediatric CNS tumors. Astrocytomas are the most common histologic type of brainstem tumor. Most brainstem gliomas are diffuse lesions, that are low signal on T1 weighted images, high signal on T2 weighted images, and have variable enhancement patterns. These tumors are usually malignant fibrillary astrocytomas (WHO grade III or IV). Some brain stem gliomas will have a focal well defined MRI appearance, and are usually lower grade (WHO grade I or II) tumors. Exophytic tumors can either grow dorsally into the fourth ventricle (usually low grade) or ventrolaterally as in this case. Usually such ventrally directed exophytic tumors are of a high histologic grade.

REFERENCE

Jallo GI, Rohrbaugh AB, Freed D. Brainstem Gliomas. *Childs Nerv Syst.* 2004;20:143–53.

CASE 5-8

A 64-year-old woman previously in good health (aside from occasional bouts of hiccup) reports the acute onset of headache, nausea, and vomiting. The symptoms are worst in the morning and appear to subside later in the day. The family doctor performs a full physical including neurological examination. No focal neurological abnormalities are found except for moderate gait ataxia and nystagmus. Fundus examination shows mild papilledema not associated with impairment of visual fields or visual acuity. A brain MRI is obtained.

Neuroimaging is shown in Figs. 5-8-1–5-8-5.

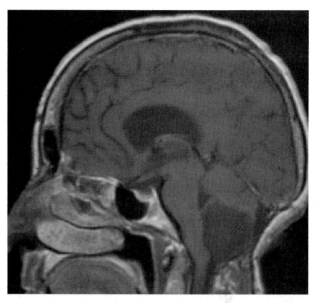

FIG. 5-8-2 Sagittal T1 MRI. This midline scan confirms that the lesion signal is slightly different from that of CSF. The lesion is located in the inferior half of the posterior fossa displacing the cerebellum upward and contacting the bulbar dorsal surface.

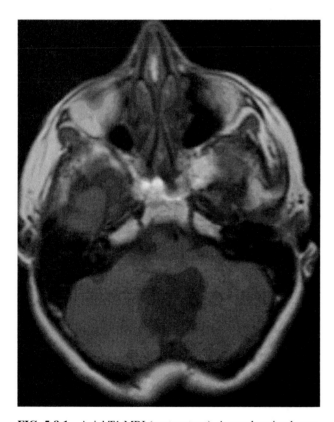

FIG. 5-8-1 Axial T1 MRI (postcontrast). A nonehancing homogeneous hypointense lesion can be appreciated in the midline of the posterior fossa. This lesion displaces laterally the cerebellar hemispheres and anteriorly the brain stem. The signal intensity is slightly higher compared with that of the CSF. Higher cuts do not show evidence of hydrocephalus.

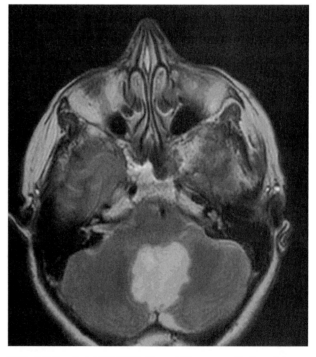

FIG. 5-8-3 Axial T2 MRI. The midline mass displays intense hyperintensity. The borders of the lesion appear to be irregular but there is no parenchymal infiltration.

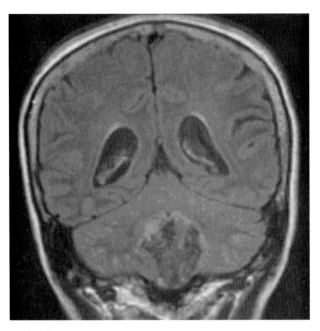

FIG. 5-8-4 Coronal proton density MRI. This examination shows that the lesion is not homogeneous. Two cystic cavities are appreciable in the superior half, divided by a band of tissue. The signal is clearly different from that displayed by the CSF in the lateral ventricles.

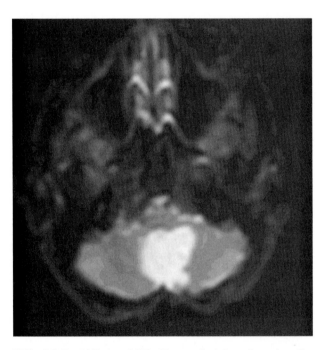

FIG. 5-8-5 Diffusion MRI. The marked hyperintensity displayed by the lesion (indicative of restricted diffusion) is helpful in the differential diagnosis from an arachnoid cyst, which would be characterized by hypointense (dark) signal.

Clinical-Radiological Diagnosis: Dermoid tumor.

KEY FACTS

The combination of low signal on T1 and high signal on T2 and diffusion scans together with absence of contrast enhancement is highly suggestive of a dermoid or epidermoid lesion. Most commonly, midline lesions are dermoids while epidermoids are more often located laterally. In this case, pathology following resection showed evidence of a dermoid lesion.

CASE 5-9

A 25-year-old woman comes to the office to see her family doctor and shows a scheduled follow-up brain MRI. She has a known history of multiple benign brain tumors requiring a series of procedures. The first procedure was performed when she was 17 years-old on a giant right petroclival neurofibroma (which was subtotally resected). After 2 years she underwent resection of a cervical neurofibroma growing mostly outside the spine on the right side. LINAC radiosurgery was then performed for a left acoustic schwannoma. A second radiosurgery was performed on a contralateral acoustic schwannoma (using a Cyberknife). The control MRI just obtained shows a new tumor originating in the 3rd ventricle and growing downward toward the interpeduncular cistern. Subsequently she is treated again with Cyberknife radiosurgery. General examination reveals severe cachexia (body weight is 45 kg for a height of 165 cm), 3 large café-au-lait spots and several skin nodules. Neurological exam is remarkable for hyperreflexia, hypophonia (following resection of the petroclival neurofibroma), peripheral facial nerve palsy, and loss of hearing on the left side (following radiosurgery).

Neuroimaging is shown in Figs. 5-9-1–5-9-4.

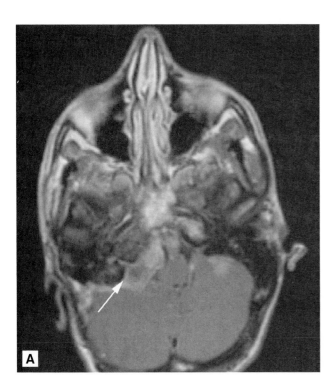
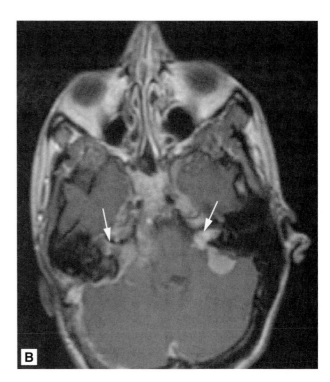

FIG. 5-9-1   Axial T1 postcontrast MRI. **A.** The arrow points to the residual right petroclival neurofibroma. The lesion has remained stable for 8 years after subtotal resection. **B.** Bilateral lesions involving the acoustic nerves (white arrows). The left neurofibroma is slightly hyperintense, a common finding following stereotactic radiosurgery.

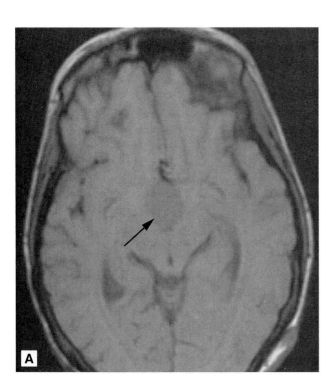
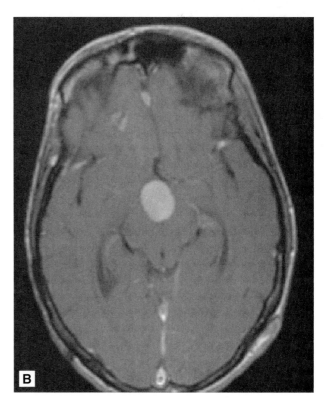

FIG. 5-9-2   **A.** Axial T1 MRI. Noncontrast MRI shows a slightly hypointense lesion compressing and displacing the surrounding brain parenchyma (black arrow). **B.** Vivid homogeneous contrast enhancement can be appreciated following intravenous injection of gadolinium.

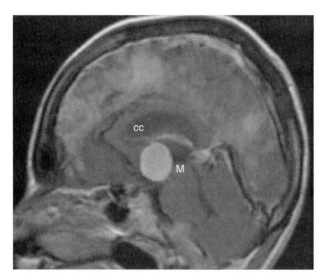

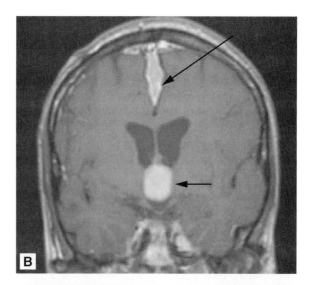

FIG. 5-9-3 Sagittal postcontrast MRI. This sagittal midline cut is remarkable for the diffuse enhancement of the falx cerebri, suggestive of a meningioma growing "en plaque" (further confirmation can be obtained looking at the coronal pictures shown subsequently). A midline contrast-enhancing lesion located in the anterior half of the 3rd ventricle between the corpus callosum (cc) and the midbrain (M) is evident. The anterior commissure is located just anterior to the tumor.

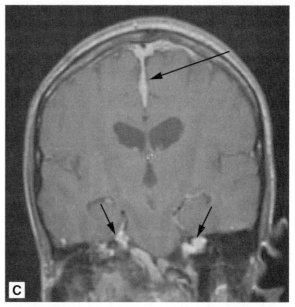

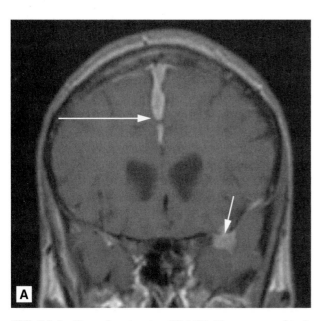

FIG. 5-9-4 Coronal postcontrast T1 MRI. The presence of multiple lesions is readily appreciated on this sequence of coronal scans. Thickening of the falx, suggestive of a meningioma "en plaque" is evident on all the scans (long arrows). Other lesions can be appreciated on the temporal side of the lesser sphenoid wing, within the 3rd ventricle, within both the acoustic pori and on the cerebellar side of the left tentorium (short arrows). *(Continued)*

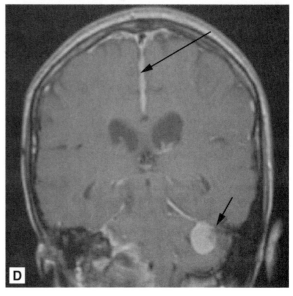

FIG. 5-9-4 *(Continued)*

Clinical-Radiological Diagnosis: Neurofibromatosis type II.

KEY FACTS

Bilateral masses involving the VIII nerve (commonly called acoustic neuromas) are pathognomonic of neurofibromatosis II (NFII), NF II, a genetic disease characterized by autosomal dominant inheritance. Patients with NFII develop early in life multiple lesions which can be characterized as neurofibromas, meningiomas, schwannomas and gliomas. The lesions seen above could be either meningiomas, neurofibromas, or schwannomas. Definitive diagnosis relies on pathology, which is not always easy or recommended to obtain. However, the avid and homogeneous contrast enhancement characterizing most of the lesions here shown is suggestive of a diagnosis of meningiomas (with the exception of the bilateral acoustic nerve lesions which are more likely to be neurofibromas or schwannomas).

CASE 5-10

A 54-year-old woman develops progressive weakness of the right leg. Neurological examination reveals spastic paresis associated with briskly increased deep tendon reflexes and ankle clonus. Increased reflexes can be found also in the left leg. No other neurological abnormalities are found.

Neuroimaging is shown in Figs. 5-10-1–5-10-2.

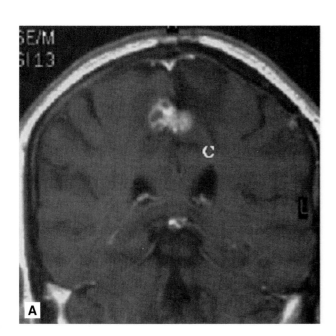
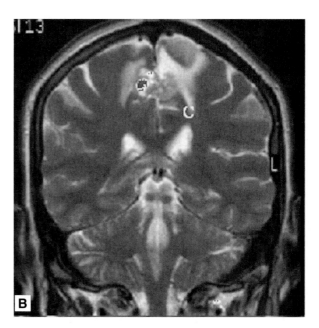

FIG. 5-10-1 Coronal T1 MRI **A.** postcontrast reveals the presence of a contrast-enhancing hyperintense lesion originating from the lower border of the falx cerebri and extending on both sides, with a larger component on the right side. The lesion is well demarkated from cerebral tissue wich is compressed and displaced. This lesion is quite heterogenous due to multiple cystic cavities. The cortex surrounding the lesion is edematous, especially on the left side, as suggested by hypointensity on T1 and hyperintensity on T2 **B.** Edema does not cross the cingulate sulcus (C) on either side.

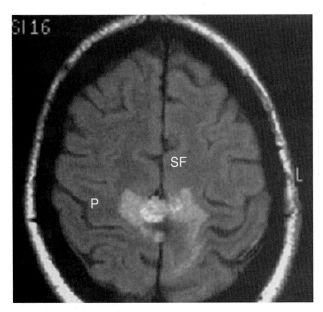

FIG. 5-10-2 An axial FLAIR shows that the edema is localized in the mesial region of the motor cortex where the somatotopic representation of the leg is usually mapped. The precentral sulcus (P) can be easily identified tracing it back from the superior frontal (SF) gyrus.

Clinical-Radiological Diagnosis: Haemangiopericytoma.

KEY FACTS

Haemangiopericytoma is a rare intracranial neoplasm usually presenting as a firm vascular tumor attached to the meninges. It is characterized by a high rate of local recurrence following resection with the possibility of extraneural metastases. Final diagnosis relies on pathology specimens but a heterogenous contrast-enhancing lesion such as the one described above is higly suggestive of haemangiopericytoma. The imaging appearance may be identical to that of a meningioma. The presence of necrosis, the lack of adjacent bony hyperostosis, and the presence of skull erosion may be distinguishing radiologic features.

CASE 5-11

Over the course of several months a 40-year-old woman develops progressive weakness in both legs, dysphonia, and dysphagia. Worsening dizziness then appears, followed by nausea and headache. Neurological examination reveals deficits of the IX-X-XI cranial nerves associated with spastic paraparesis and mild papilledema. Brain MRI shows evidence of a non-contrast enhancing bulbar lesion growing exophytically. A diagnosis of pilocytic astrocytoma (WHO grade I) is made based on a surgical specimen. The lesion is then treated by Cyberknife radiosurgery delivering 21 Gy in 3 fractions of 7 Gy each. The treatment plan (based on a T2 MRI) is shown in Fig. 5-11-1 and illustrates well the compression exerted by the tumor on the bulb which is displaced anteriorly and compressed against the clivus, assuming a crescentic shape and a hypointense signal due to edema.

After radiosurgery, the patient is followed with serial MRI scans revealing radio-induced edema which appears approximately 6 months after the treatment and resolves after 15 months. A course of steroids has been necessary during this period. The patient receives a follow-up MRI 24 months after the treatment. At this time most of the symptoms previously described (paraparesis, dysphonia, dysphagia) have partially improved.

Neuroimaging is shown in Figs. 5-11-1–5-11-3.

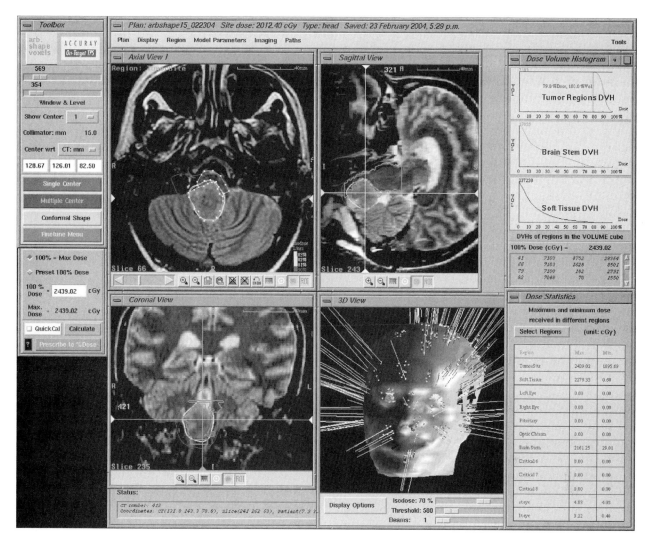

FIG. 5-11-1   Treatment plan.

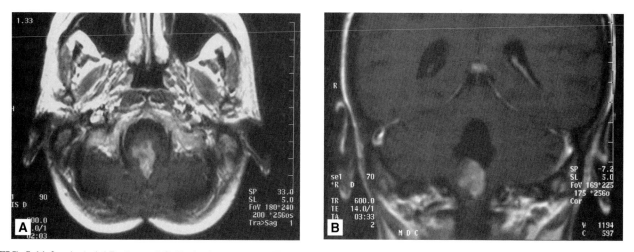

FIG. 5-11-2   A. Axial **B.** Coronal **C.** Sagittal postcontrast T1 MR. An irregularly shaped hyperintense noncontrast enhancing lesion posterior to the bulb can be appreciated. The lesion is much smaller than the one immediately before treatment. The brainstem is quite decompressed and does not touch the clivus anymore. *(Continued)*

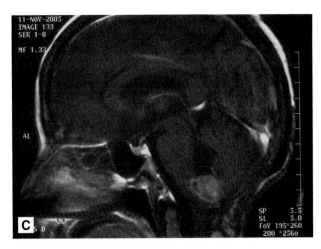

FIG. 5-11-2 *(Continued)*

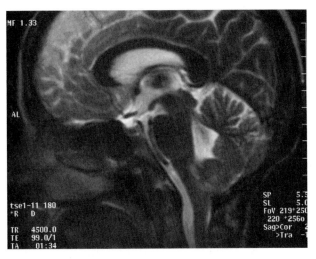

FIG. 5-11-3 Sagittal T2 MRI. The lesion is mostly hypointense to the brain with some scattered areas of hyperintensity.

Clinical-Radiological Diagnosis: Pilocytic glioma regression following radiosurgery.

KEY FACTS

Radiosurgery is an emerging therapeutic modality developed initially for the treatment of selected brain lesions. Arrays of beams delivered stereotactically to the target can induce tumor necrosis while the surrounding tissue may develop radio-induced edema. This

case gives a good example of tumor regression following radiosurgery. This pilocytic astrocytoma is smaller and develops a heterogeneous hyperintense signal on T1 scans without contrast enhancement.

CASE 5-12

A 36-year-old woman presents with chronic headaches and the recent onset of mild left hemiparesis (noticed upon neurological examination by slight drift of upper and lower extremities with eyes closed).

Neuroimaging is shown in Figs. 5-12-1–5-12-2.

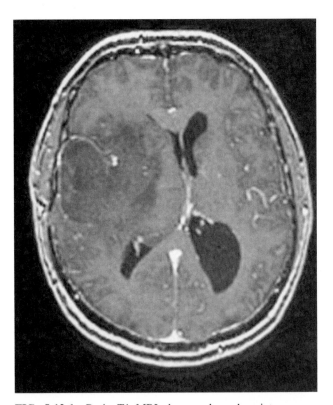

FIG. 5-12-1 Brain T1 MRI shows a large hypointense area involving the right insula and temporal lobe. No contrast enhancement can be appreciated. The signal within the lesion is moderately heterogeneous. Some degree of midline shift is present. The lateral ventricles are compressed and displaced toward the midline on the right side and enlarged on the left side.

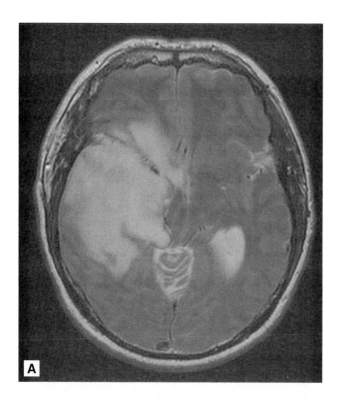

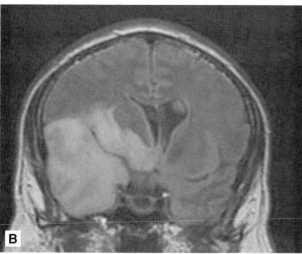

FIG. 5-12-2 **A.** T2 axial and **B.** coronal MRIs provide excellent definition of the gross boundaries of this large lesion. The lesion is hyperintense and displays a homogeneous high signal involving the right anterior temporal lobe, insula, and the mesial and basal part of the frontal lobe. The basal ganglia are displaced but not infiltrated by this lesion.

Clinical-Radiological-Pathological Diagnosis: Diffuse glioma. Pathology after subtotal resection revealed a grade II diffuse glioma.

KEY FACTS

Low grade gliomas will often have infiltrative growth patterns that do not disrupt the blood brain barrier, and therefore will not enhance after contrast administration. It is important to note that though these tumors have a better prognosis than anaplastic astrocytomas (WHO grade III) and glioblastoma multiforme (grade IV), they can undergo malignant degeneration and transform into a higher grade tumor.

CASE 5-13

A 56-year-old man with a history of well controlled epilepsy presented to the emergency room with over 1 hour of seizures involving his right upper extremity. In the past, the patient's typical seizures had always affected the left upper extremity. MRI revealed a new lesion with significant edema in the left temporal lobe. Resection confirmed the diagnosis of glioblastoma multiforme.

Neuroimaging is shown in Fig. 5-13-1.

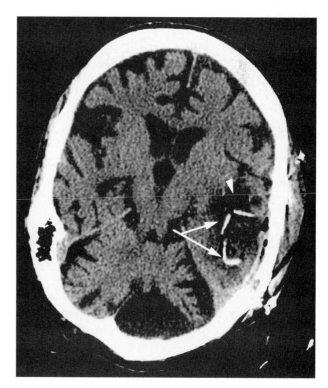

FIG. 5-13-1 This CAT scan image was acquired 2 days postresection. Postoperative changes include the hyperdense bars (white arrows). These are carmustine (BCNU) containing wafers (Gliadel) placed at the resection edge. Additionally, some air (arrowhead) is present within the temporal lobe. The large fluid filled space adjacent to the left cerebellum is long standing.

Clinical-Radiological Diagnosis: Postoperative changes with small residual tumor.

KEY FACTS

A significant change in a patient's usual seizure type should always be thoroughly evaluated. Iatrogenic etiologies of abnormal neuroimaging findings should always be considered in the postoperative patient.

CASE 5-14

A 54-year-old man undergoes radical resection of a cervical spine intraaxial lesion. A pathological diagnosis of ependymoma is made. A scheduled follow-up brain and spine MRI is performed 3 months after surgery.

  Neuroimaging is shown in Figs. 5-14-1–5-14-2.

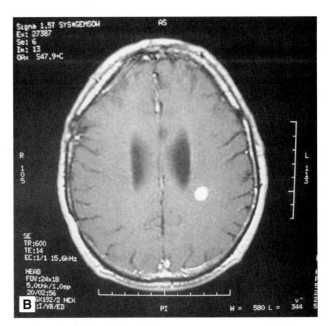

FIG. 5-14-1   B. The lesion shows avid homogeneous enhancement following contrast injection.

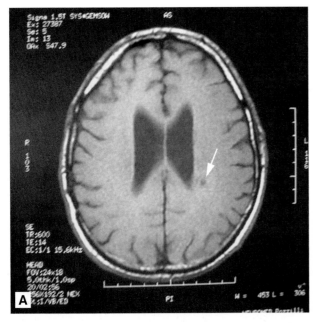

FIG. 5-14-1   A. Axial noncontrast T1 MRI shows a small rounded hypointense lesion in the white matter of the central compartment of the left hemisphere (white arrow).

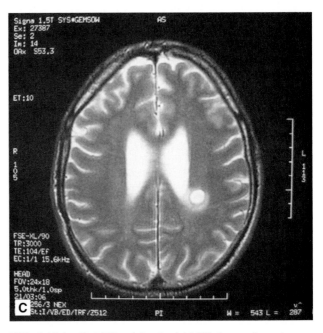

FIG. 5-14-1   C. A T2 weighted axial MRI shows a hyperintense homogeneous lesion surrounded by a halo of high signal suggesting local edema.

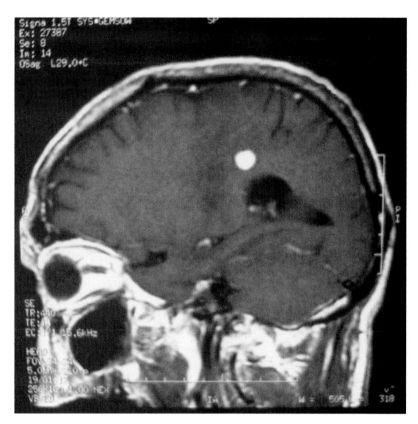

FIG. 5-14-2 This parasagittal post-contrast T1 MRI shows that the lesion is close but not adjacent to the roof of the right lateral ventricle.

Clinical-Radiological Diagnosis: Metastatic ependymoma.

KEY FACTS

Ependymomas can easily spread through CSF pathways and produce distant localizations. Most common are drop metastases down in the spine. This is a rare case of supratentorial metastatic localization. This lesion was treated with radiosurgery after a stereotactic brain biopsy. Supratentorial ependymomas will often calcify. Infratentorial ependymomas are usually in the fourth ventricle and grow out the foramen of Magendie and Luschka, with a plastic, toothpaste appearance.

CASE 5-15

An 11-year-old boy with a history of a tumor involving the left temporal lobe, status post resection 1 year ago now presents with headaches and intermittent emesis. The patient has had radiation treatment post operatively.

Neuroimaging is shown in Figs. 5-15-1–5-15-4.

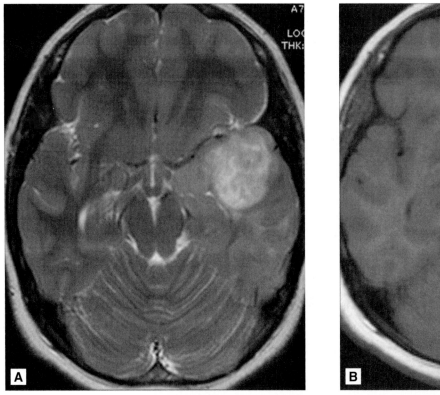
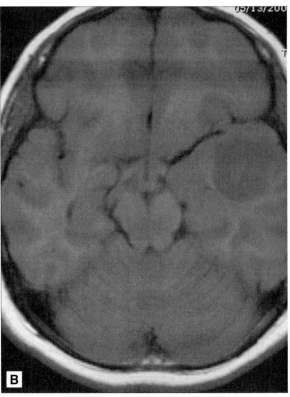

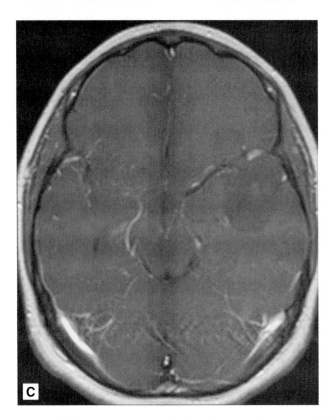

FIG. 5-15-1   The patient's initial presenting MRI scan shows a lesion in the left temporal lobe. **A.** Axial T2 weighted MRI images show a high signal intensity lesion in the left temporal lobe. **B.** There is a corresponding low T1 signal intensity lesion. **C.** There is faint central enhancement on post gadolinium T1 weighted images. The imaging appearance of the initial lesion is not specific. The differential diagnosis of a supratentorial intraaxial lesion includes an astrocytoma, an atypical teratoid rhabdoid tumor, an oligodendroglioma, or an ependymoma. If this lesion was extraaxial, it could represent a meningioma.

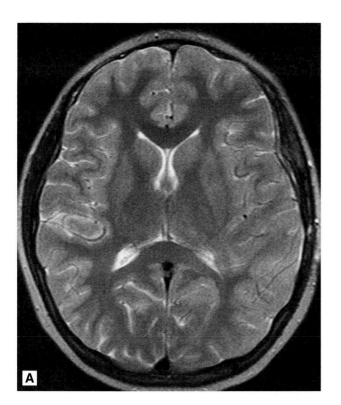

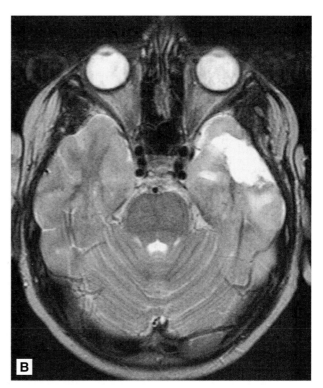

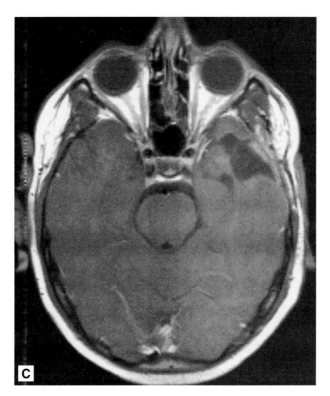

FIG. 5-15-2 **A.** An MRI study after resection of the tumor shows the left basal ganglia to be normal in appearance. Axial T2 weighted image (B), and post gadolinium T1 weighted image (C) shows a normal post resection cavity without evidence of enhancement.

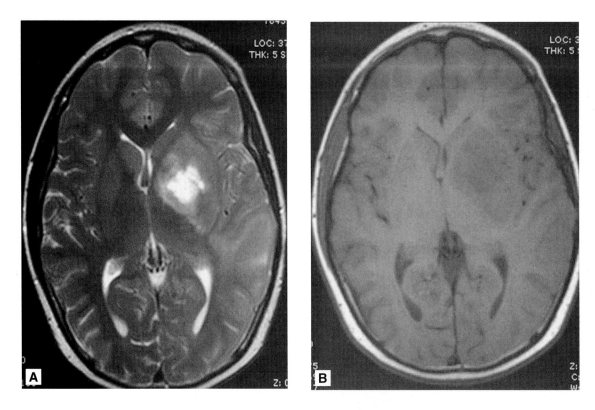

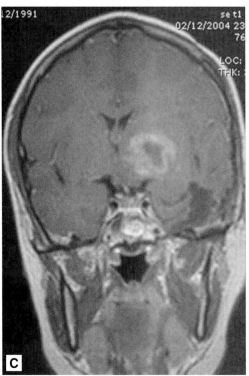

FIG. 5-15-3 Axial T2 weighted image (A), precontrast T1 weighted image (B), and a coronal post gadolinium T1 weighted image (C) show a necrotic mass lesion in the left basal ganglia, with peripheral ring enhancement. The differential diagnosis of this lesion includes radiation necrosis or tumor recurrence.

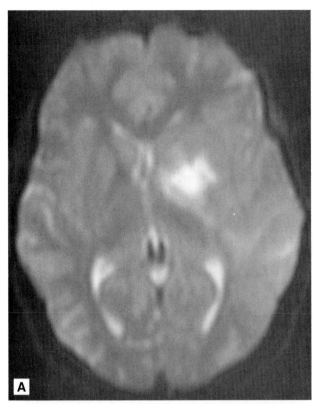

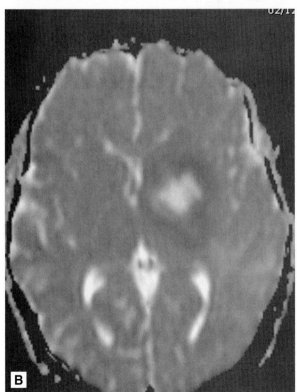

FIG. 5-15-4 **A.** Diffusion weighted image and **B.** The apparent diffusion coefficient map (ADC) show a centrally necrotic lesion, with restricted peripheral diffusion, shown as a dark region on the ADC map. These findings are consistent with recurrent tumor in the left basal ganglia.

Clinical-Radiological Diagnosis: Recurrent supratentorial primitive neuroectodermal tumor.

KEY FACTS

Supratentorial primitive neuroectodermal tumors are highly cellular tumors that account for 2.5–6% of pediatric brain tumors. They are histologically related to medulloblastomas, pineoblastomas, atypical teratoid rhabdoid tumors, and neuroblastomas. The MRI appearance includes heterogenous enhancement, usually with a sharply marginated mass. These tumors can be found in the ventricles or in the cerebral hemisphere. They can have areas of necrosis or calcification. Embryonal tumors such as PNET, malignant teratoid rhabdoid, and medulloblastomas have restricted diffusion compared to low grade gliomas and non-embryonal high grade gliomas, thought to be due to the highly cellular nature of these tumors.

REFERENCES

Barkovich JA. Intracranial, orbital, and neck masses of childhood. in: *Pediatric Neuroimaging.* Lippincott Williams and Wilkins. 2005;507–658.

Gauvain K, McKinstry RC, Mukherjee P et al. Evaluating pediatric brain tumor cellularity with diffusion tensor imaging. *Am J Rosentgenol.* 2001;177:449–54.

CASE 5-16

A 15-month-old child presents with nausea, vomiting, unsteady gait, and lethargy.

Neuroimaging is shown in Figs. 5-16-1–5-16-2.

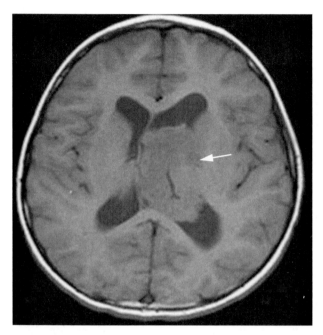

FIG. 5-16-1 Precontrast T1 weighted image shows a lobulated, frond like mass lesion in the left lateral ventricle which is isointense to grey matter (white arrow). The left lateral ventricle is slightly expanded compared to the right lateral ventricle.

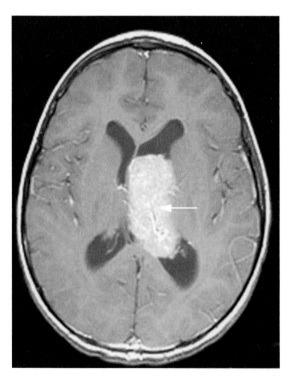

FIG. 5-16-2 Postcontrast T1 weighted image shows this mass to enhance homogenously (white arrow).

Clinical-Radiological Diagnosis: Choroid plexus papilloma.

KEY FACTS

Choroid plexus papillomas are rare intracranial neoplasms, usually found in children, often in the first 2 years of life. In children they occur in the lateral ventricles, usually in the atria. In adults they are found in the fourth ventricle. They can be found in the third ventricle or be multifocal. CT may show calcification. On MRI they are isointense to hypointense masses on T1 and isointense to hyperintense masses on T2. On both CT and MRI these lesions show homogenous enhancement. Usually they are histologically benign. These tumors are hypervascular by angiography.

Case courtesy of Jordan Rosenblum, MD

REFERENCES

Coates TL, Hinshaw DB, Peckman N, et al. Pediatric choroid plexus neoplasms: MR, CT, and pathologic correlation. Radiology. 1989;173:81–88.
Osborn Anne G. *Diagnostic Imaging: Brain.* 60th ed. Salt Lake City, Utah: Amirsys; 2004:1–6.

CASE 5-17

A 50-year-old man presented with headaches and intermittent episodes of dizziness.
Neuroimaging is shown in Figs. 5-17-1–5-17-3.

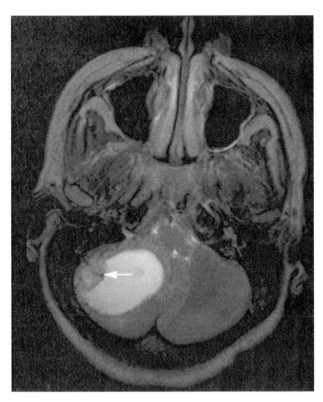

FIG. 5-17-1 Precontrast T1 weighted image shows a predominantly cystic mass in the right cerebellum with a solid nodule in the right lateral aspect of the cystic component (white arrow). There is mass effect on the pons and cerebellum.

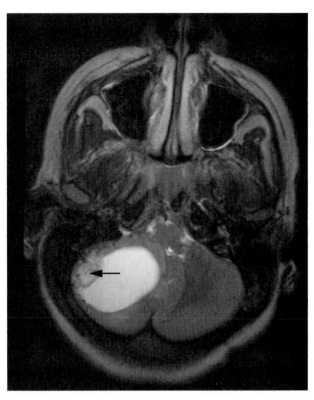

FIG. 5-17-3 T2 weighted image shows the nodule slightly iso to hyperintense to grey matter. The cystic component is better demonstrated on T2 weighted images.

Clinical-Radiological Diagnosis: Hemangioblastoma.

KEY FACTS

Hemangioblastomas are benign neoplasms of endothelial origin that can occur sporadically or in association with Von Hippel Lindau disease (4–20%). They are the most common infratentorial tumors of adult patients and are characterized by a hypervascular mural nodule that abuts the pia. In addition to the cerebellum these tumors can be found in the spine, brainstem, and cerebrum. On MRI these lesions most commonly are cystic lesions with a hypervascular mural nodule. They can be solid tumors with or without a central cystic region. Treatment is surgical resection, sometimes with preoperative embolization.

Case courtesy of Jordan Rosenblum, MD

REFERENCES

Lee SR, Saches J, Mark AS, Dillon WP, et al. Posterior fossa hemangioblastomas: MR imaging. *Radiology.* 1989;171: 463–68.
Choyke PL, Glenn GM, McClellan WM, et al. B. von Hippel Lindau Disease: Genetic, Clinical, and Imaging Features.

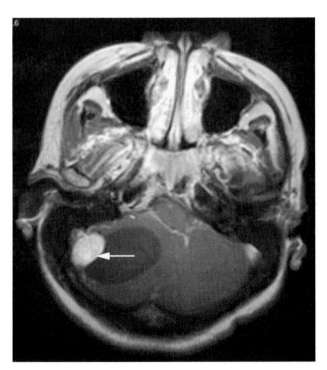

FIG. 5-17-2 Postcontrast T1 weighted image shows the mural nodule to enhance avidly (white arrow).

CASE 5-18

A 30-year-old woman presents with a history of menstrual cycle irregularities, vaginal dryness, and loss of libido. Her pertinent laboratory findings include a prolactin level of 250 µg/mL.

Neuroimaging is shown in Figs. 5-18-1–5-18-3.

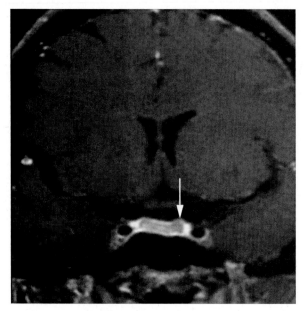

FIG. 5-18-1 Pituitary microadenoma. Post gadolinium T1 weighted images show a low signal intensity region in the left side of the pituitary gland, with an associated focal contour deformity.

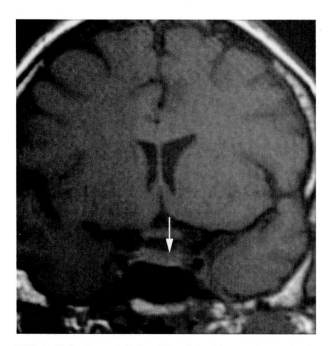

FIG. 5-18-2 Pre gadolinium T1 weighted images do not clearly demonstrate a pituitary lesion.

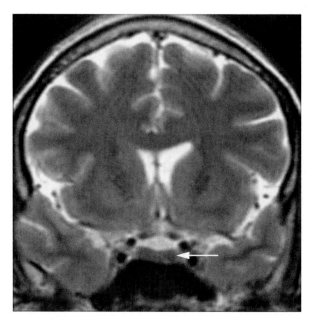

FIG. 5-18-3 On coronal T2 weighted images there is an area of low signal within the left side of the gland suggestive of a small adenoma more clearly demonstrated after gadolinium administration.

Clinical-Radiological Diagnosis: Pituitary microadenoma

KEY FACTS

Pituitary adenomas are the most common lesion in the sella, accounting for 10–15% of all intracranial tumors. Lesions less than 10mm are called microadenomas. Lesions greater than 10 mm are macroadenomas. Lesions less than 3 mm are usually adrenocorticotropic hormone (ACTH) producing adenomas. Microadenomas are often an incidental finding (6–27%).

Microadenomas are usually hypointense on precontrast T1 weighted images, and may have variable signal intensity on T2 weighted images. Deviation of the pituitary stalk has a wide range of normal variation and is difficult to use as a diagnostic sign. Dynamic contrast enhanced images increase the sensitivity of microadenoma detection. Delayed post contrast images (> 20 minutes) may show increased enhancement within the lesion.

The most common endocrinologically active pituitary adenomas are prolactinomas. A serum prolactin level above 200 µg/L is very specific for an adenoma. Growth hormone producing adenomas can produce acromegaly in adults and gigantism in children. ACTH producing adenomas cause Cushing disease.

REFERENCES

Bonneville JF, Bonneville F, Cattin F. Magnetic resonance imaging of pituitary adenomas. *Eur Radiol.* 2005;15:543–48.

Balagura S, Frantz AG, Housepian EM, Carmel PW. The specificity of serum prolactin as a diagnostic indicator of pituitary adenoma. *J Neurosurg.* 1979;51:42–6.

Lum C, Kucharcyzk W, Montanera WJ, et al. The Sella Turcica and Parasellar Region. In: *Magnetic Resonance Imaging of the Brain and Spine*. Atlas S (ed.), Philadelphia PA. Lippincott Williams and Wilkins, 2002;1283–1362.

Simard MF. Pituitary tumor endocrinopathies and their endocrine evaluation. *Neurosurg Clin N Am*. 2003;14:41–54.

Teramoto A, Hirakawa K, Sanno N, Osamura RY. Incidental pituitary lesions in 1000 unselected autopsy specimens. *Radiology*. 1994;193:161–4.

CASE 5-19

A 43-year-old man is evaluated by an ophthalmologist for a swollen eye associated with ocular pain. Symptoms started over 1 year ago and progressed slowly. The patient denies visual dysfunction. Physical examination reveals chemosis and proptosis of the right eye. Visual field testing reveals a concentric restriction while visual acuity is grossly preserved. The range of eye movements is not affected. Pupillary size is larger compared to the contralateral eye. Pupillary response to light is sluggish but present.

Neuroimaging is shown in Figs. 5-19-1–5-19-3.

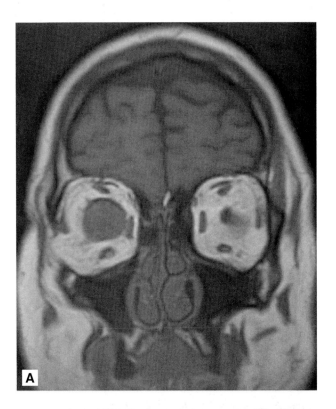

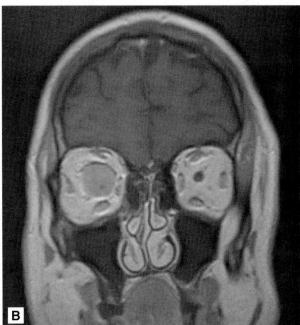

FIG. 5-19-2 Coronal pre- **A.** and postcontrast **B.** cuts show the avid contrast enhancement following gadolinium injection . On the post-contrast coronal cut, the optic nerve can be easily appreciated as a dark, hypointense circle within the bright, hyperintense lesion and, again, is characterized by a smaller size compared to the opposite nerve. The extraocular mucles are easily appreciated on coronal cuts.

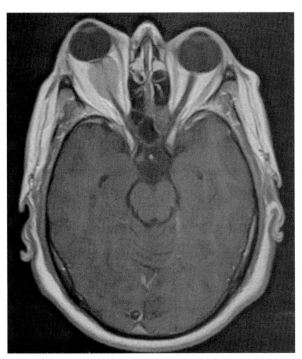

FIG. 5-19-1 Axial brain MRI reveals the presence of a homogeneously enhancing lesion located in the ocular cavity. A conic mass with base located anteriorly and pushing forward the ocular globe. The ocular globe itself is slightly deformed but no structural abnormalities can be appreciated within the lens and the anterior and posterior chamber. The right optic nerve can be identified as a tiny hypointense signal centrally located and surrounded by hyperintense contrast-enhancing tissue. Comparison with the contralateral optic nerve shows that the affected right optic nerve is markedly atrophic.

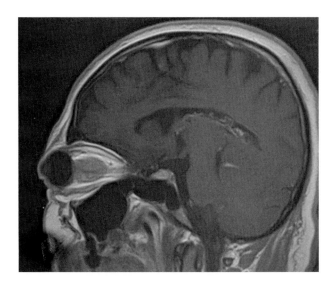

FIG. 5-19-3   Postcontrast sagittal brain MRI.

Clinical-Radiological Diagnosis: Optic nerve sheath meningioma.

KEY FACTS

A slowly growing, contrast-enhancing lesion pushing anteriorly on the ocular globe with concentric restriction of visual fields but without gross failure of the visual acuity during early stages is likely to be an optic nerve sheath meningioma. Optic nerve gliomas are characterized by faster onset of loss of vision while the structure of the nerve cannot be distinguished and contrast enhancement can be absent or inhomogeneous. Granulomas can occasionally grow in the optic cavity but are usually in a more peripheral location and do not display the homogeneous enhancement typical of meningiomas.

CASE 5-20

A 72-year-old man presents with headache and recent onset of double vision. Neurological exammination shows inability to externally rotate the right eye, suggesting a right VI nerve palsy. Fundoscopic examination is normal.

Neuroimaging is shown in Fig. 5-20-1.

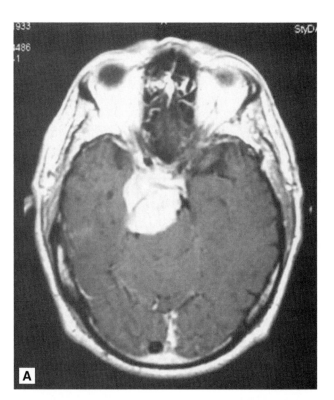

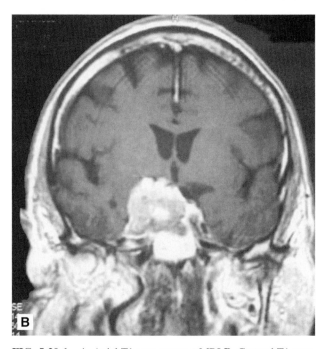

FIG. 5-20-1   A. Axial T1 postconstrast MRI **B.** Coronal T1 post-contrast MRI. Brain T1 weighted MRI post-contrast shows a right-sided petroclival contrast enhancing mass causing compression and distortion of the anterior surface of the pons. This lesion also grows in the middle fossa invading the homolateral cavernous sinus. No other gross abnormalities can be appreciated and the size of the ventricles is not enlarged **C.** Sagittal T1 post-contrast MRI.
(Continued)

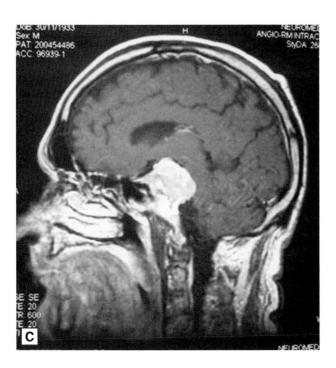

FIG. 5-20-1 *(Continued)*

Clinical-Radiological Diagnosis: Petroclival meningioma.

KEY FACTS

The clinical presentation of this lesion is a focal neurological sign: this fact, together with the absence of signs of raised intracranial pressure, strongly suggests that this is a slowly growing lesion. Homolateral sixth nerve palsy is caused by the stretching of this long nerve originating from the dorsal surface of the brainstem and travelling along the longest intracranial pathway among the cranial nerves.

Chapter 6

TRAUMA

CASE 6-1

An 18-year-old man was hit in the head with a baseball bat. Neuroimaging is shown in Fig. 6-1-1.

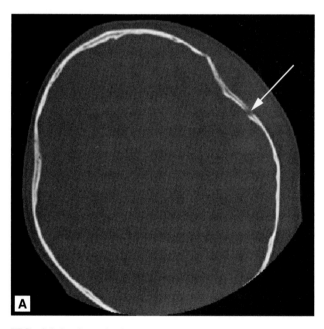

FIG. 6-1-1 **A.** Axial images with bone windows show a fracture of the squamous portion of the left temporal bone **B.** There is an underlying crescentic biconvex fluid collection, high attenuation along its more posterior aspect, and mixed attenuation along its anterior aspect. The hematoma is restricted by the cranial suture lines anteriorly and posteriorly. The hyperattenuating clot and swirling lucency seen in the anterior aspect represents acute blood. *(Continued)*

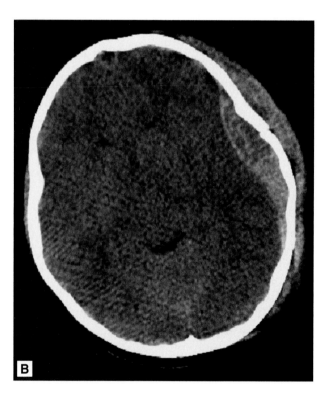

FIG. 6-1-1 *(Continued)*

Clinical-Radiological Diagnosis: Epidural hematoma.

KEY FACTS

Epidural hematomas commonly occur in association with temporal bone fractures because the middle meningeal artery is lacerated. Epidural hematomas can also occur from a laceration of a dural sinus.

CASE 6-2

A 21-year-old man was punched in the left eye during a bar fight.

Neuroimaging is shown in Figs. 6-2-1–6-2-3.

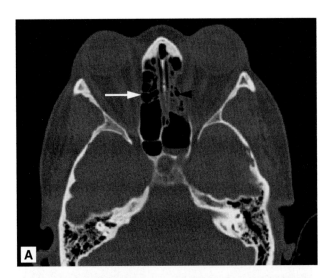

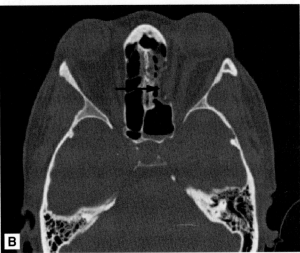

FIG. 6-2-1 **A** and **B.** Axial images with bone windows show the normal medial wall of the right orbit (white arrow). There is fluid (black arrowhead) in the left ethmoid air cells. There is a fracture of the medial wall of the left orbit (black arrow).

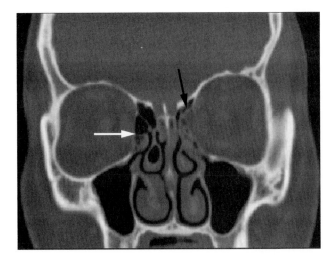

FIG. 6-2-2 Coronal reconstructions again demonstrate the normal medial wall of the right orbit (white arrow). There is fluid in the left ethmoid air cells along with an associated fracture of the medial wall of the left orbit (black arrow).

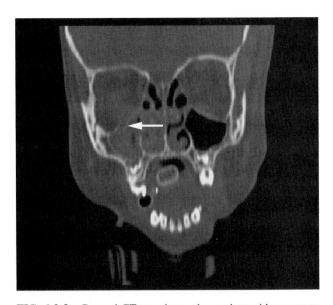

FIG. 6-2-3 Coronal CT scan in another patient with trauma to the right orbit demonstrates a fracture of the floor of the right orbit (white arrow). The most common locations for an orbital blowout fracture are the floor and the medial wall of the orbit.

Clinical-Radiological Diagnosis: Orbit fracture.

KEY FACTS

Blunt trauma to the eye can result in "blowout" fractures of the medial wall (lamina papyracea of the ethmoid bone) or the inferior wall (floor) of the orbit. The presence of air in the orbit, fluid in the adjacent involved sinus, and adjacent soft tissue swelling are all indirect signs of an orbital fracture.

CASE 6-3

A 56-year-old man is found lying on the floor by his son. He is minimally responsive and brought to the emergency room. Apparently he had been involved in some type of altercation at a local bar the evening before. Head CT was performed 4 days following the fight.

Neuroimaging is shown in Figs. 6-3-1–6-3-2.

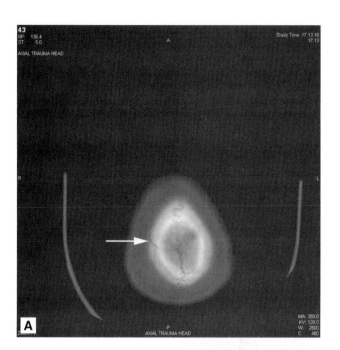
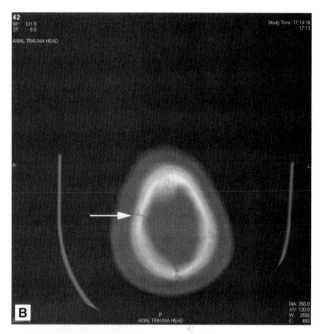
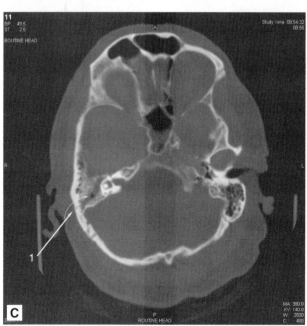

FIG. 6-3-1 A, B, and **C.** Bone windows demonstrating a right parietal and longitudinal right temporal bone fracture extending through auditory canal (1).

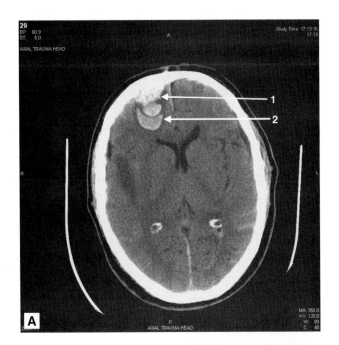

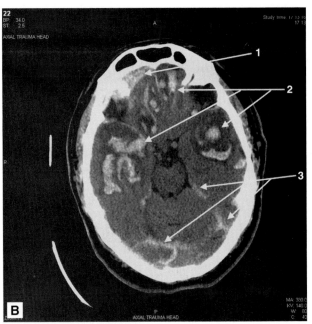

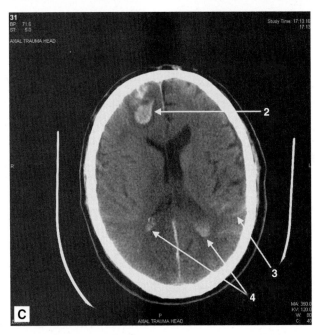

FIG. 6-3-2   A, B, C. Right frontal subdural (1) and multiple intraparenchymal (2) hematomas. There is edema surrounding the intraparenchymal hemorrhages with a small amount of mass effect as evidenced by distortion of the right lateral ventricle. Scattered subarachnoid blood is present bilaterally (3), as well as intraventricular hemorrhage (4).

Clinical-Radiological Diagnosis: Multiple hemorrhages and fractures following head trauma.

KEY FACTS

Brain hemorrhages following trauma will often evolve over the first 24–72 hours.

INFECTIONS

CASE 7-1

A 50-year-old man presents with endocarditis, stiff neck, fevers, and altered mental status.

Neuroimaging is shown in Figs. 7-1-1–7-1-2.

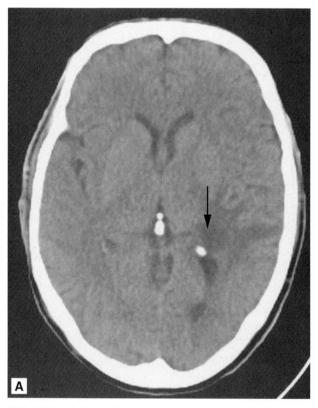

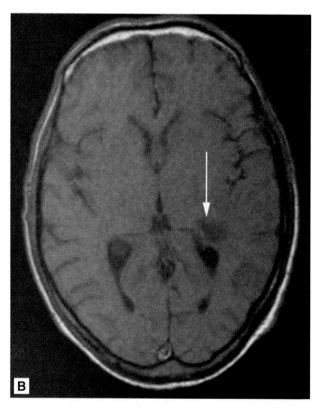

FIG. 7-1-1 **A.** Head CT shows a low attenuation region (black arrow) in the left periventricular white matter. **B.** Precontrast T1 weighted images show the corresponding area to have low signal intensity (white arrow). **C.** After contrast administration, this region (white arrowhead) shows ring enhancement. In addition there is abnormal enhancement in the frontal horn of the left lateral ventricle (white arrow). *(Continued)*

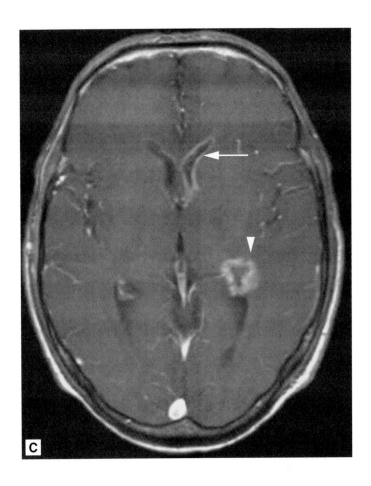

FIG. 7-1-1 *(Continued)*

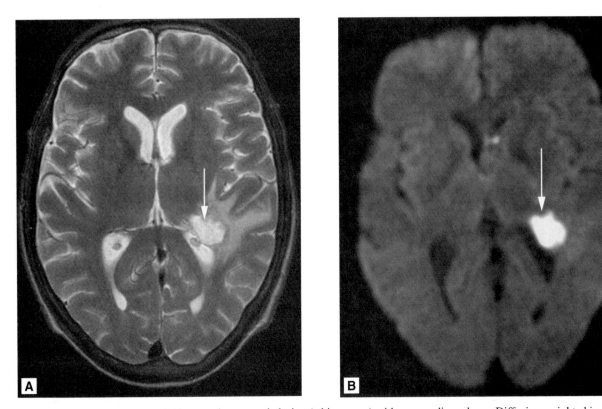

FIG. 7-1-2 (A) T2 weighted axial images show a cystic lesion (white arrow) with surrounding edema. Diffusion weighted images (B) and the apparent diffusion coefficient map (C) shows restricted diffusion within the lesion (white arrow). *(Continued)*

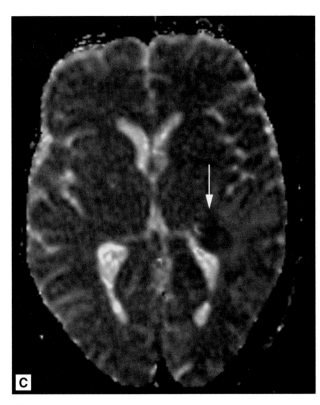

FIG. 7-1-2 *(Continued)*

Clinical-Radiological Diagnosis: Abscess with ventriculitis.

KEY FACTS

A brain abscess will be high signal intensity on T2 weighted images, low signal on T1 weighted images, and will show ring enhancement after contrast administration. The imaging features can make the distinction from a cystic or necrotic tumor difficult. Diffusion weighted imaging will show restriction in brain abscesses, which can often help in making this distinction.

REFERENCE

Guo AC, Provenzale JM, Cruz LCH, et al. Cerebral abscesses: investigation using apparent diffusion coefficient maps. *Neuroradiology.* 2001;43:370–4.

CASE 7-2

A 43-year-old man presented to the emergency room, 2 hours following an apparently unprovoked generalized tonic clonic seizure. He is a little sleepy, but otherwise examination is normal. The patient emigrated from El Salvador 14 years ago, and has not been outside of the United States in over 6 years.

Neuroimaging is shown in Figs. 7-2-1–7-2-2.

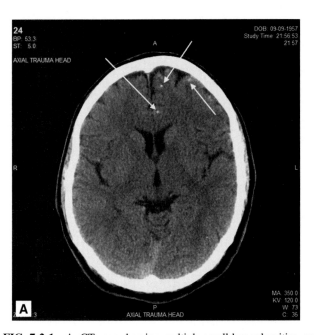
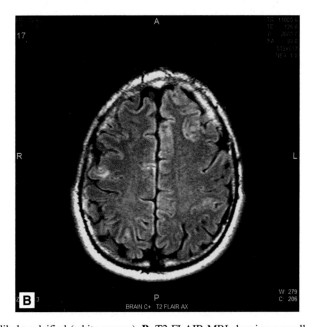

FIG. 7-2-1   A. CT scan showing multiple small hyperdensities, some likely calcified (white arrows). **B.** T2 FLAIR MRI showing a small lesion in the posterior right frontal lobe, with a central area of low signal and surrounding edema. **C.** The central portion of the right frontal lesion also has low T1 signal suggesting calcification. **D.** Ring-enhancing lesions (white arrows) indicating some degree of active disease. *(Continued)*

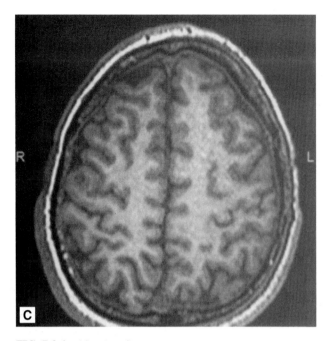

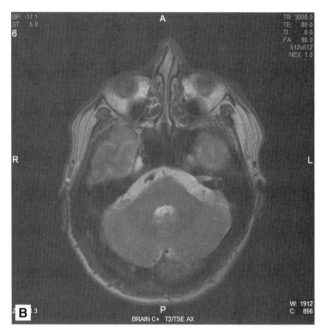

FIG. 7-2-1 *(Continued)*

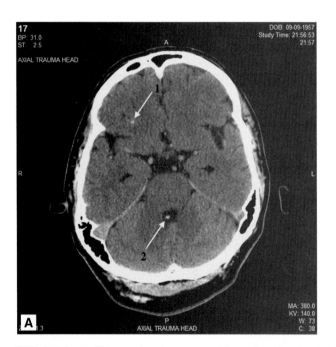

FIG. 7-2-2   A. CT scan showing two small hyperdensities. Lesion (2) is possibly the parasite scolex. **B** and **C.** T2 and T1 MRIs showing what may be the partially developed parasite within the fourth ventricle (alternatively this may be prominent calcified choroid plexus). **D.** After contrast there is partial enhancement of the lesion. *(Continued)*

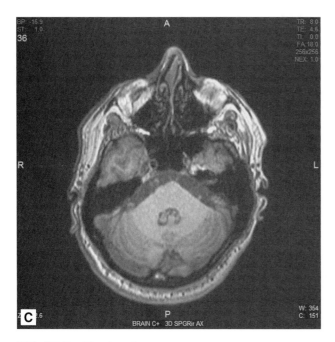

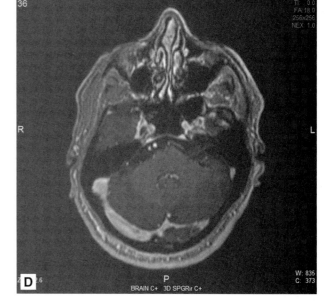

FIG. 7-2-2   *(Continued)*

Clinical-Radiological Diagnosis: Neurocysticercosis at various stages of manifestation. This patient likely acquired the disease within the United States.

KEY FACTS

The exact time course and pathophysiology of the disease are somewhat speculative. Neurocysticercosis has three active (vesicular, colloidal, and granular) and one inactive (nodular) stage(s). The active phases are characterized by cysts, edema, and contrast enhancement. The nodular stage is characterized by 2–10 mm calcifications, often better seen on CT. Some calcified lesions may also show contrast enhancement or edema.

REFERENCE

Castillo, M. Imaging of neurocysticercosis. *Semin Roentgenol.* 2004;6(7):465–73.

Chapter 8

MULTIPLE SCLEROSIS AND AUTOIMMUNE DISORDERS

CASE 8-1

A 43-year-old woman originally presented at age 30 with blurring of vision in the right eye. This resolved nearly completely within one month, but in the years since, she has had various transient neurological symptoms, including urinary incontinence, weakness, and sensory dysfunction.

Neuroimaging is shown in Figs. 8-1-1–8-1-2.

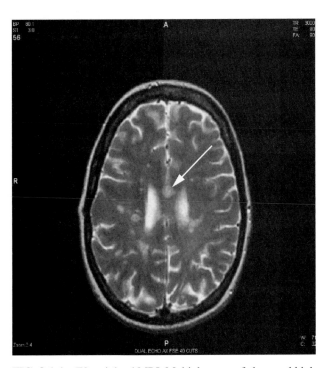

FIG. 8-1-1 T2 weighted MRI. Multiple areas of abnormal high signal are scattered throughout the white matter of both hemispheres. The arrow points to a lesion in the corpus callosum. The pattern is typical, but not diagnostic of that which occurs in multiple sclerosis or acute demyelinating encephalomyelitis.

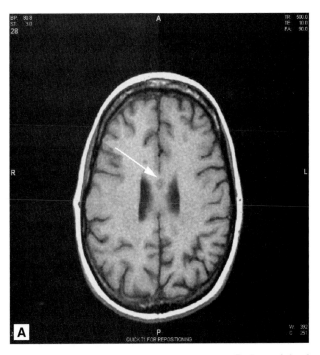

FIG. 8-1-2 **A.** T1 weighted MRI precontrast. **B.** T1 weighted MRI postcontrast demonstrating that the corpus callosal lesion is enhancing (Fig. 8-1-1). *(Continued)*

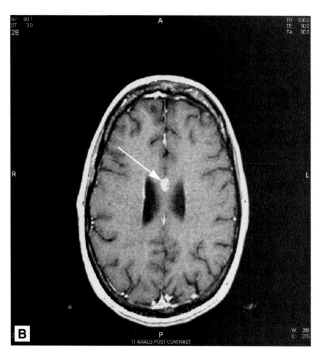

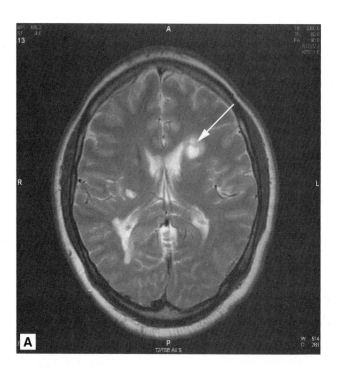

FIG. 8-1-2   *(Continued)*

Clinical-Radiological Diagnosis: Multiple sclerosis.

KEY FACTS

Since one lesion enhanced but others did not, it suggests that both a chronic and active disease process is occurring. Multiple sclerosis is characterized by multiple lesions in space and time.

CASE 8-2

A 32-year-old man, who had emigrated from Bolivia 3 years ago, awoke one week ago with a tingling sensation in his left neck. Over the course of the next 1–2 days it progressed to involve his entire left body and extremities from the neck down. He then developed clumsiness and weakness of the left hand as well as difficulty walking. He tried some sort of herbal treatment for 2 days with no effect and came in to the emergency room. Examination findings included left upper and bilateral lower extremity dysmetria (L>R). There was an upper motor neuron pattern of weakness in the left upper and lower extremity (distal>proximal).

Neuroimaging is shown in Figs. 8-2-1–8-2-3.

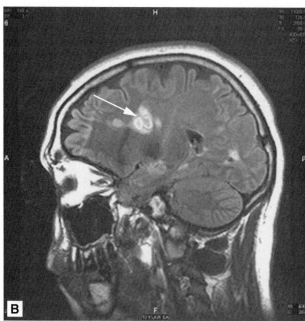

FIG. 8-2-1   A. T2 axial. **B.** T2 FLAIR sagittal sequences demonstrating multiple areas of abnormal high signal. The largest lesion (arrow) has a lamellar appearance.

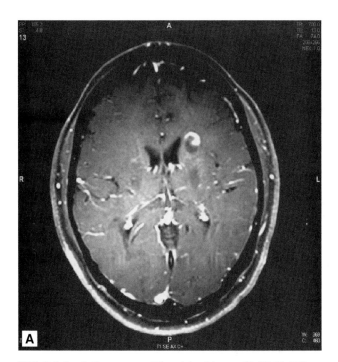
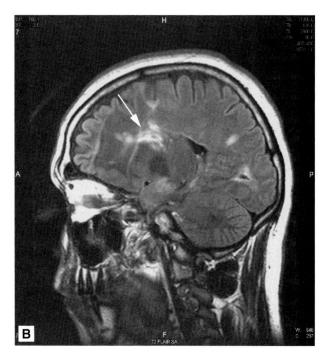

FIG. 8-2-2   A. Postcontrast T1 weighted image. **B.** T2 FLAIR sequence show enhancement along part of the border of the largest lesion.

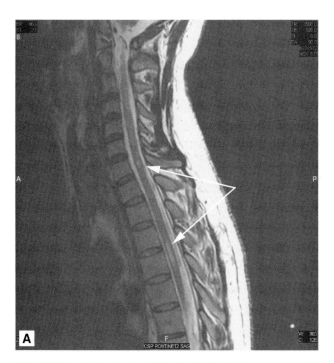
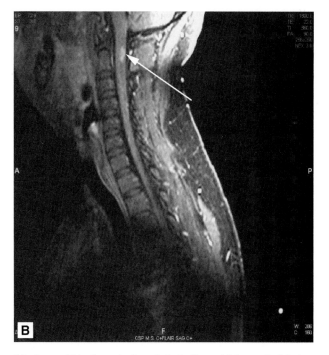

FIG. 8-2-3   A. Postcontrast T2. **B.** T2 FLAIR images revealed several lesions within the spinal cord, including a high cervical lesion likely responsible for the presenting symptoms.

Clinical-Radiological Diagnosis: Acute disseminated encephalomyelitis with a high likelihood of progressing to clinically definite multiple sclerosis. Additionally, the images are consistent with a rare type demyelinating disease known as Baló's concentric sclerosis.

KEY FACTS

Baló's concentric sclerosis had traditionally been thought to have a very poor prognosis, but more recent evidence indicates that the finding is not predictive of clinical outcome.

Chapter 9

VASCULAR LESIONS

CASE 9-1

The patient is a 52-year-old woman with sudden onset of headaches, nausea, vomiting, and photophobia on the morning of admission.

Neuroimaging is shown in Figs. 9-1-1–9-1-3.

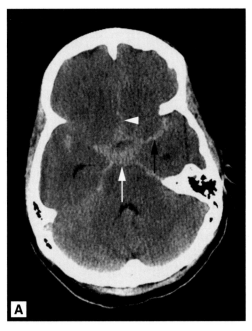 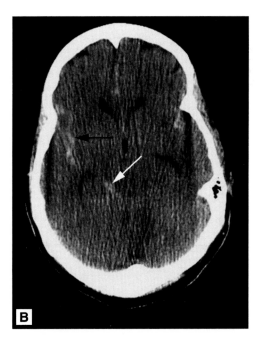

FIG. 9-1-1 A. Head CT on admission shows blood in the basilar cistern (white arrow), in the left sylvian fissure (black arrow) and in the anterior interhemispheric fissure (white arrowhead). **B.** Head CT on admission also shows blood in the right sylvian fissure (black arrow) and the right ambient cistern (white arrow).

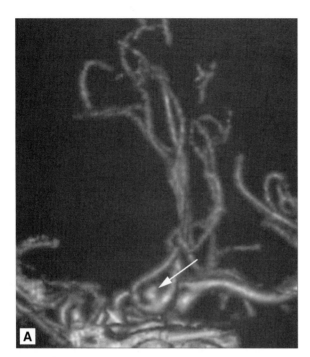 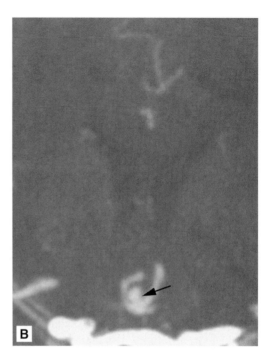

FIG. 9-1-2 **A.** A 3-D reconstruction of a CT angiogram shows a small aneurysm of the anterior communicating artery (white arrow). **B.** The aneurysm is also seen on the coronal slab maximum intensity projection images (black arrow).

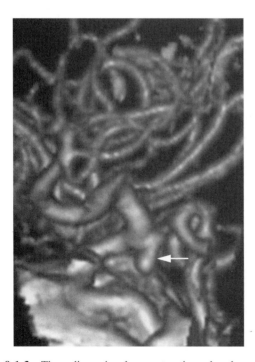

FIG. 9-1-3 Three dimensional reconstructions also show a left posterior communicating artery aneurysm (white arrow).

Clinical-Radiological Diagnosis: Aneurysmal subarachnoid hemorrhage.

KEY FACTS

In the absence of trauma the most common cause of subarachnoid hemorrhage is a ruptured aneurysm. The most common locations of aneurysms are the anterior communicating artery, the supraclinoid internal carotid artery (including the posterior communicating artery), the middle cerebral artery, and the basilar artery.

Though angiography is still the gold standard for aneurysm detection, CT angiography has emerged as a very sensitive noninvasive method to detect aneurysms. With the advent of three dimensional angiography technology, angiography often provides anatomic details that are useful in developing a treatment strategy (endovascular coiling versus surgical clipping).

CASE 9-2

The patient is a 14-year-old girl who presented with headaches, nausea, and vomiting while running on a

treadmill. On presentation in the ER the patient had neck stiffness, and photophobia, but was otherwise neurologically intact.

Neuroimaging is shown in Figs. 9-2-1–9-2-3.

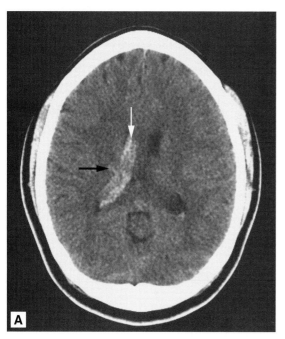
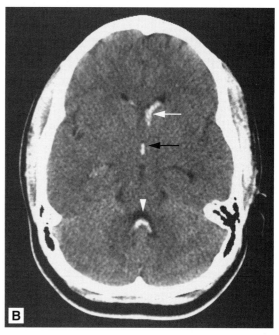

FIG. 9-2-1 **A.** Initial noncontrast head CT at the time of presentation shows casting blood in the right lateral ventricle (white arrow), with a small adjacent intraparenchymal focus (black arrow). **B.** There is casting blood in the left lateral ventricle (white arrow), third ventricle (black arrow), and fourth ventricle (white arrowhead).

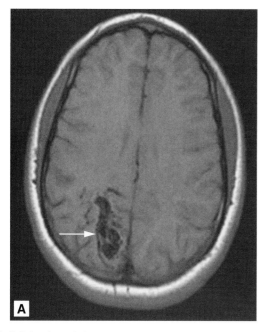
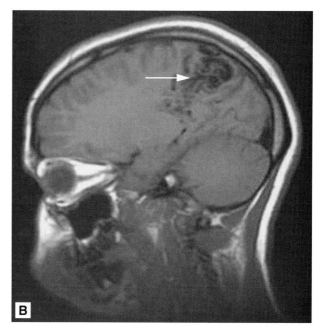

FIG. 9-2-2 **A.** Axial pre-contrast T1 weighted image shows serpiginous flow voids in the right parietal region (white arrow). **B.** It is important to note on the sagittal image that the lesion is superior to the parieto-occipital sulcus, and thus would not be expected to affect the patient's vision.

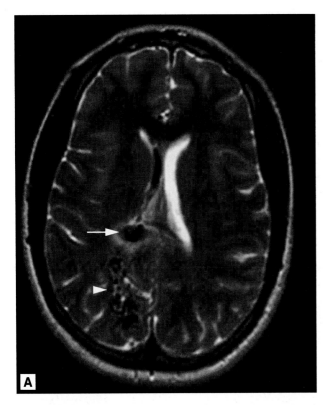 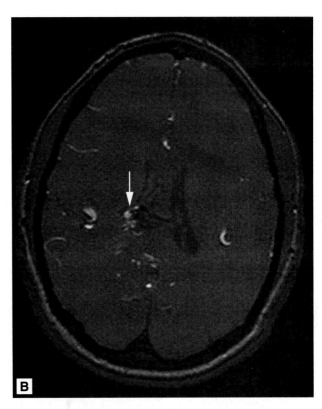

FIG. 9-2-3 **A.** Axial T2 weighted images show dark signal, representing hemorrhage in the right lateral ventricle and in the adjacent parenchyma (white arrow). There are serpiginous flow voids in the right parietal region (white arrowhead), representing an arteriovenous malformation. **B.** Source image from an MR angiogram shows a distal feeding vessel flow related aneurysm (white arrow).

Clinical-Radiological Diagnosis: Arteriovenous malformation with intraventricular hemorrhage.

KEY FACTS

An arteriovenous malformation (AVM) is an abnormal connection between arteries and veins with an intervening nidus, without a normal capillary bed. These lesions can present as an intraparenchymal or intraventricular hemorrhage, with seizures, headaches, or in children with headaches or hydrocephalus.

An intraventricular hemorrhage usually arises as an extension of an intraparenchymal hemorrhage, often in older patients from an extension of a deep hypertensive hemorrhage. In young adults and teenagers, a ruptured arteriovenous malformation is the most common cause. Pure intraventricular hemorrhages can arise from an aneurysm (particularly 4th ventricle hemorrhages from a ruptured PICA aneurysm), AVM, or tumor. AVMs can have an aneurysm within the nidus itself, on the feeding artery, or along a draining vein. In addition, patients with an AVM are more likely to have an aneurysm on a vessel that is unrelated to the AVM.

CASE 9-3

The patient is a 16-year-old boy who has a history of a severe headache after a wrestling match. Head CT performed at an outside hospital showed a hemorrhage. The patient's neurologic examination was normal. EEG was unremarkable.

Neuroimaging is shown in Figs. 9-3-1–9-3-2.

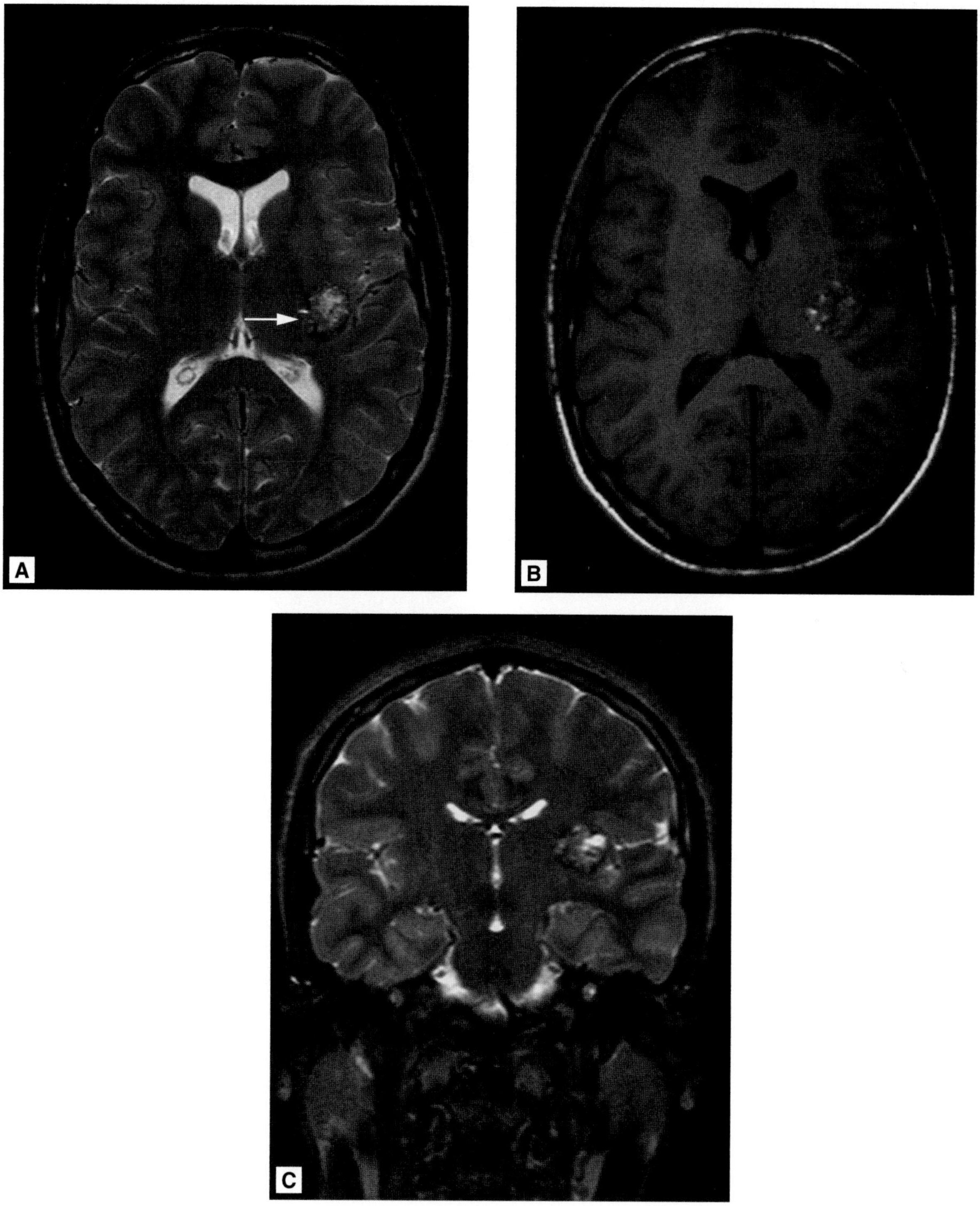

FIG. 9-3-1 **A.** Axial T2 weighted image shows a lesion along the posterior aspect of the left putamen, with central punctuate areas of high signal, and a surrounding low signal region, in a characteristic popcorn appearance (white arrow). **B.** Axial T1 weighted image shows punctuate areas of high signal. **C.** Coronal T2 weighted image also demonstrates a characteristic popcorn lesion with punctate areas of high signal centrally and a surrounding low signal rim.

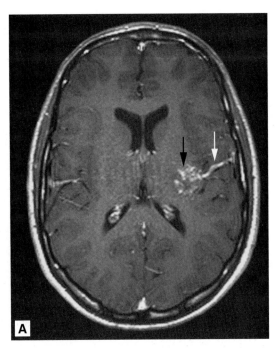 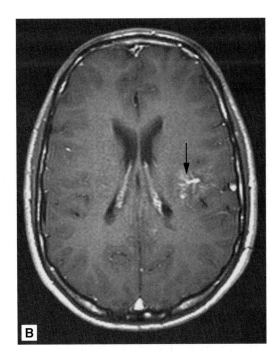

FIG. 9-3-2   **A** and **B.** Axial postcontrast T1 weighted images show a draining vein (white arrow) with a caput medusae pattern (black arrow) adjacent to the cavernoma.

Clinical-Radiological Diagnosis: Cavernoma with an associated developmental venous anomaly.

KEY FACTS

A cavernoma is a benign vascular lesion, consisting of a well-defined collection of endothelium-lined vessels. Clinically these lesions can present with seizures, headaches, an intraparenchymal hemorrhage, or focal neurological deficits. Often patients will be asymptomatic at presentation. Cavernomas are seen on CT scans as an area of high attenuation, with Hounsfield units consistent with either hemorrhage or calcification. They classically have a popcorn appearance on T2 weighted images, and show blooming on gradient echo T2* weighted images. Cavernomas may enhance after contrast administration.

A developmental venous anomaly can be associated with cavernomas. These are the most common vascular malformation in the central nervous system (CNS), and have a "caput medusae" appearance. It is important to keep in mind that these lesions drain normal brain parenchyma.

CASE 9-4

A 30-year-old healthy woman, taking oral contraceptives, with no other significant past medical history presents with subacute onset of headaches over the past two weeks, with an acute worsening of her headache as well as nausea and vomiting on the day of admission. On examination the patient has left upper extremity weakness, but is otherwise neurologically intact.

Neuroimaging is shown in Figs. 9-4-1–9-4-4.

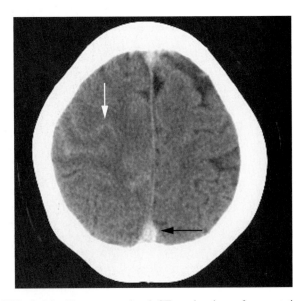

FIG. 9-4-1   Non-contrast head CT at the time of presentation demonstrates subarachnoid blood over the right cerebral convexity (white arrow). The surrounding brain parenchyma is edematous. On non-contrast views, the superior sagittal sinus appears expanded and is of abnormally high attenuation, worrisome for sinus thrombosis (black arrow). This is known as the dense cord sign.

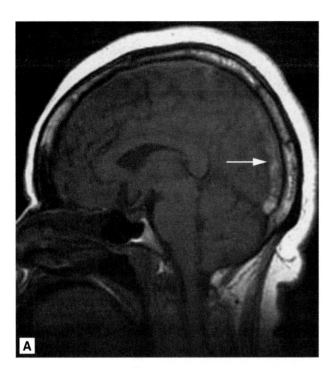

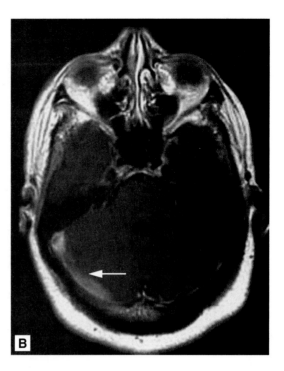

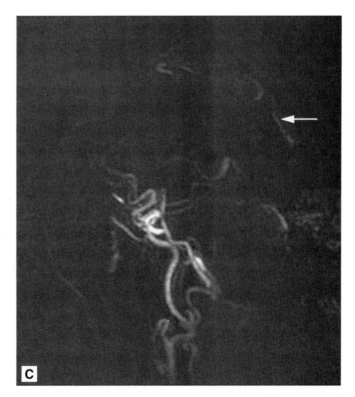

FIG. 9-4-2 **A.** Sagittal pre-contrast T1 weighted MRI scan shows increased signal within the superior sagittal sinus. This represents thrombus within the superior sagittal sinus (white arrow). **B.** Axial pre-contrast T1 weighted image shows abnormal high signal within the right transverse sinus, also consistent with thrombosis (white arrow). **C.** MR Venogram using a phase contrast technique does not demonstrate a normal sagittal sinus (white arrow).

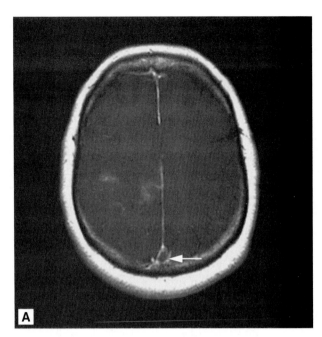

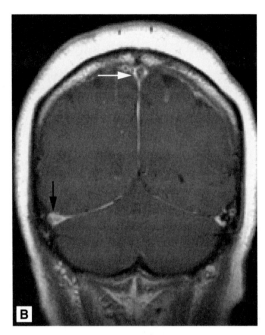

FIG. 9-4-3 **A.** Axial and coronal **B.** post gadolinium T1 weighted images show thrombus within the superior sagittal sinus. This pattern of a filling defect within the superior sagittal sinus is called a delta sign (white arrow). The lack of enhancement in the right transverse sinus is seen well on coronal post gadolinium T1 weighted images (black arrow).

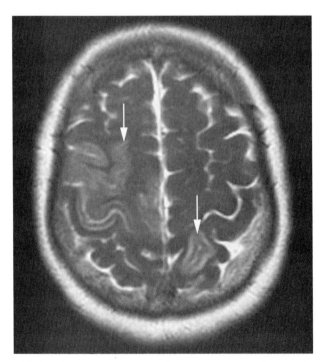

FIG. 9-4-4 Axial T2 weighted images show areas of vasogenic edema in the right frontal and left parietal lobes (white arrows).

Clinical-Radiological Diagnosis: Sagittal and right transverse sinus thrombosis.

KEY FACTS

Depending on age, blood products can have variable signal on MRI. Acute blood is isointense on T1 weighted images and hypointense on T2 weighted images. Subacute blood products will be bright on T1 weighted images. Subacute blood products may be low or high intensity on T2 weighted images. Chronic hemorrhage will demonstrate low signal on T1 and T2 weighted images. On contrast enhanced CT and MRI images, lack of enhancement in a sinus can indicate thrombosis.

On T2 weighted images one may see a lack of normal flow voids. On noncontrast head CT signs of venous thrombosis include the dense cord sign (high signal on non-contrast images), venous infarcts, slit like ventricles, and subarachnoid hemorrhage. MRI and CT venography are powerful techniques for examining the venous sinus system. Angiography remains the gold standard for deomonstrating sinus thrombosis.

CASE 9-5

A 43-year-old woman has headaches that wake her from sleep, nausea, and vomiting. On examination the patient has nuchal rigidity and photophobia. She is otherwise alert oriented, and follows commands without focal neurologic deficits.

Neuroimaging is shown in Figs. 9-5-1–9-5-2.

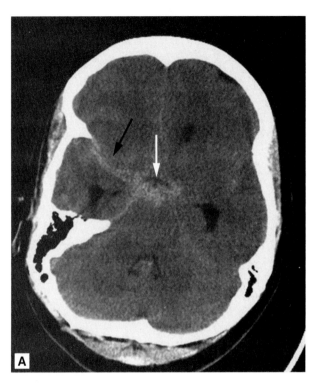
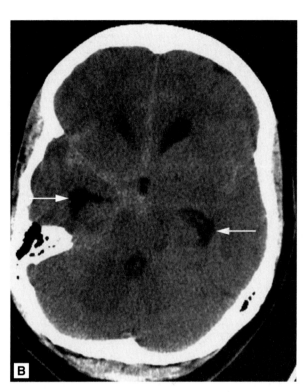

FIG. 9-5-1 **A.** The patient's initial head CT shows subarachnoid blood in the basal cistern (white arrow), as well as in the right sylvian fissure (black arrow). **B.** There is also a small amount of blood in the left sylvian fissure . The temporal horns of the lateral ventricles are dilated (white arrows).

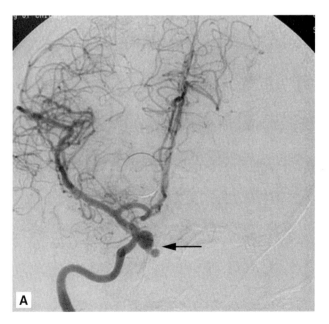
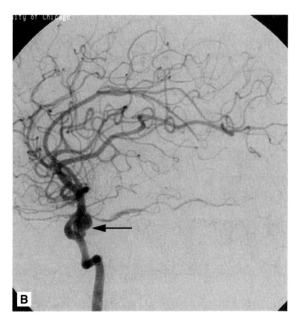

FIG. 9-5-2 The patient's angiogram shows a medially directed paraclinoid aneurysm (black arrow), with a focal tubular excrescence on the AP (A) and lateral injection (B) of the right internal carotid artery. Post coiling angiogram through the right internal carotid artery shows no aneurysm filling (C and D). *(Continued)*

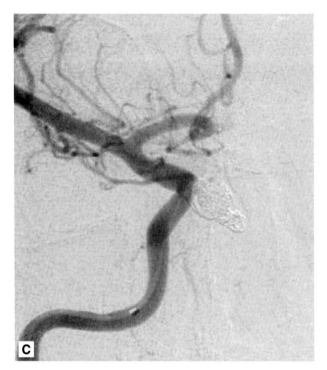

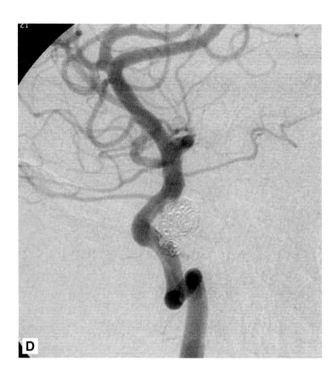

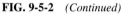

FIG. 9-5-2 *(Continued)*

Clinical-Radiological Diagnosis: Aneurysmal subarachnoid hemorrhage.

KEY FACTS

Subarachnoid hemorrhage can occur from many causes. In the absence of trauma, the most common cause is a ruptured aneurysm. Other causes include arteriovenous malformations, moya-moya disease, vasculitis, anticoagulated state, arterial dissection, venous thrombosis, or perimesencephalic nonaneurysmal subarachnoid hemorrhage.

The most common locations for an aneurysm are anterior communicating artery, middle cerebral artery bifurcation, posterior communicating artery, and basilar tip. The Fisher scale for the evaluation of subarachnoid hemorrhage is predictive of the risk of vasospasm, based on the initial non contrast head CT. Ruptured aneurysms should be treated by endovascular or surgical means within 24–48 hours of presentation. Patients with subarachnoid hemorrhage can develop hydrocephalus. Also late in the first week and in the early second week they can develop cerebral vasospasm.

CASE 9-6

The patient is a 60-year-old woman with pulsatile tinnitus in her right ear.

Neuroimaging is shown in Figs. 9-6-1–9-6-2.

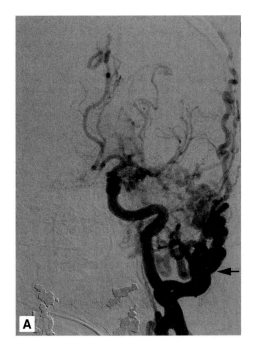
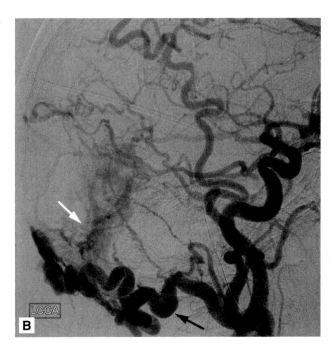

FIG. 9-6-1 A conventional angiogram with AP (A) and lateral (B) projections of a left common carotid artery injection shows in the arterial phase abnormally enlarged branches of the left external carotid artery, primarily the occipital artery (black arrow), with transosseous feeders (white arrow).

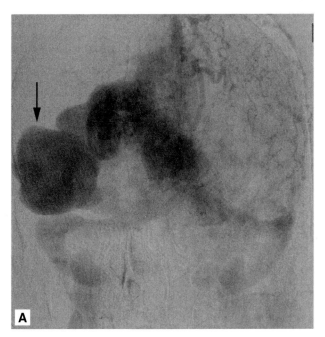
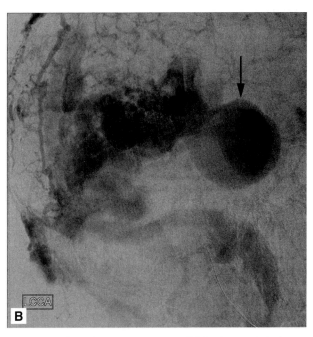

FIG. 9-6-2 Later images in the AP (A) and lateral (B) planes from the same run show the transosseous arterial feeders to drain into a markedly aneurysmally dilated deep draining vein, likely the right basal vein of Rosenthal (black arrow).

Clinical-Radiological Diagnosis: Dural arteriovenous malformation.

KEY FACTS

Dural arteriovenous fistulas are classically thought to be acquired lesions caused by sinus thrombosis of a transverse sinus, and subsequent recanalization by recruitment of external carotid artery feeders. They are abnormal arteriovenous connections lying within in the dura, with arterial supply from branches of the external carotid artery. Venous drainage can be into a sinus, or into cortical veins.

CASE 9-7

The patient is a 62-year-old woman with a history of diabetes and hypertension, who was found comatose at home by her daughter. On admission to an outside hospital she opened her eyes to painful stimulation, did not follow commands, flexed all extremities to pain, and had incomprehensible speech. Her cranial nerves were intact.

The patient was transferred after placement of a ventriculostomy catheter for further management after the outside hospital head CT showed intraventricular blood.

Neourimaging is shown in Figs. 9-7-1–9-7-8.

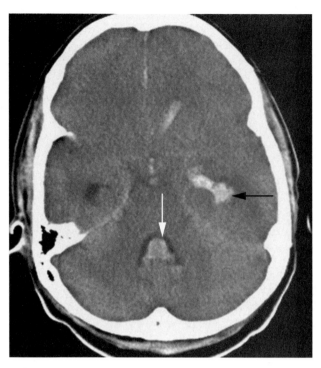

FIG. 9-7-2 A slightly higher slice from the initial noncontrast head CT after the patient was transferred shows blood in the temporal horn of the left lateral ventricle with surrounding edema (black arrow) and some intraparenchymal blood. There is again seen blood within the fourth ventricle (white arrow).

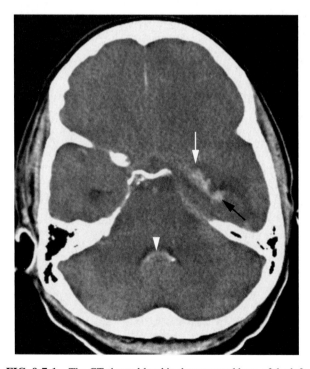

FIG. 9-7-1 The CT shows blood in the temporal horn of the left lateral ventricle (black arrow) with surrounding edema as well as some adjacent intraparenchymal blood (white arrow). Note the blood in the fourth ventricle (white arrowhead).

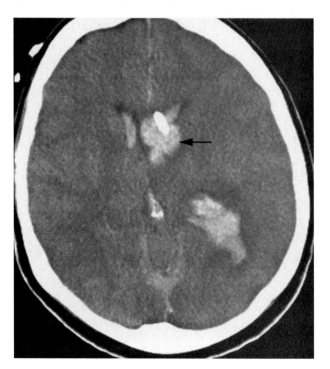

FIG. 9-7-3 On the initial head CT after transfer a small amount of intraparenchymal blood is seen in the left caudate head (black arrow), however it is in proximity to the tip of the ventriculostomy catheter.

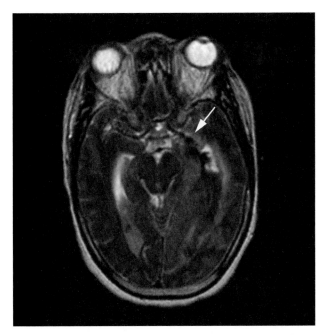

FIG. 9-7-4 Axial T2 weighted image from the patient's MRI scan show an aneurysm from the distal ICA directed toward the left temporal horn of the lateral ventricle (white arrow).

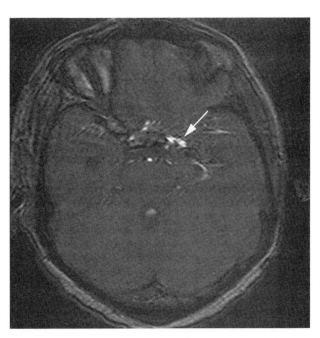

FIG. 9-7-6 Source images from the MRA also show the aneurysm to be directed posteriorly towards the temporal horn of the left lateral ventricle (white arrow).

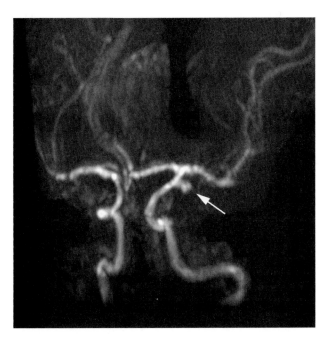

FIG. 9-7-5 Maximum intensity projection image from the MRA also demonstrates a distal left internal carotid artery aneurysm (white arrow).

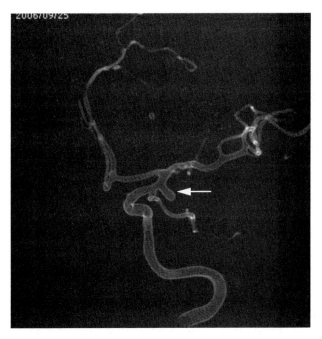

FIG. 9-7-7 Three dimentional reconstructed images from a conventional angiogram confirm the presence of an aneurysm (white arrow), distinct from the posterior communicating artery origin.

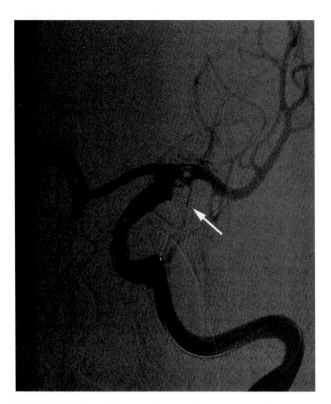

FIG. 9-7-8 Post coiling angiogram shows near complete occlusion of the aneurysm post procedure (white arrow).

Clinical-Radiological   Diagnosis: Intraventricular hemorrhage from a ruptured aneurysm.

KEY FACTS

Potential causes for an intraventricular hemorrhage are extension from an intraparenchymal hemorrhage, aneurysm rupture, AVM rupture, tumor, or vertebral artery dissection. Intraventricular hemorrhage from a ruptured aneurysm has a poor prognosis (mortality 64%).

REFERENCES

Greenberg MS. *Handbook of Neurosurgery.* New York: Thieme; 2001;177–896.

Mohr G, Ferguson G, Khan M, et al. Intraventricular hemorrhage from ruptured aneurysm. Retrospective analysis of 91 cases. *J Neurosurg.* 1983;58:482–7.

Chapter 10

EPILEPSY

CASE 10-1

A 12-year-old girl presented with a gradual progression of symptoms over the past 5 days. She first noticed intermittent tingling in her left lower extremity, which soon became accompanied by twitches. In

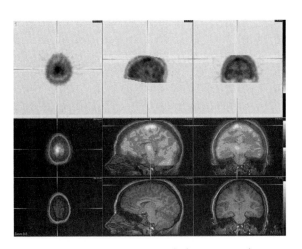

FIG. 10-1-1 Ictal single-photon emission computed tomography (SPECT) scan superimposed on MRI. The radiotracer was injected during one of the patient's clinical events. There is a clear area of increased tracer uptake in the right frontal-parietal region near the midline. This finding is supportive of the diagnosis of partial onset of seizure.

between episodes, the left lower extremity had residual weakness, which resulted in tripping and falling. By the time of presentation, the episodes were spreading to involve the entire left body. Episodes lasted approximately 2–3 minutes and were occurring up to 30 times per day. The frequency and severity of the attacks were reduced by anti-convulsant medication. EEG was normal during the events.

Neuroimaging is shown in Fig. 10-1-1.

Clinical-Radiological Diagnosis: Epilepsy partialis continua.

KEY FACTS

The coregistration of MRI with SPECT or positrom emission tomography (PET) allows relatively high-resolution structural and functional brain imaging.

CASE 10-2

The patient is a 5-year-old boy with seizures.

Neuroimaging is shown in Fig. 10-2-1.

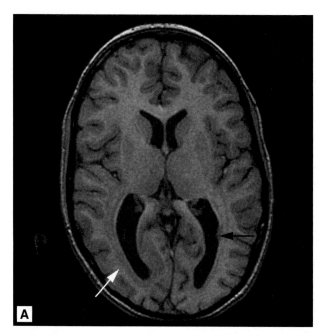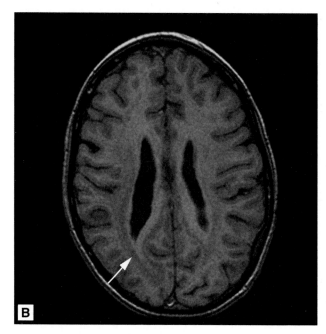

FIG. 10-2-1   **A.** Axial T1 weighted images show abnormal grey matter in a band like distribution around both lateral ventricles (white arrow). There is also a focal lesion in the occipital horn of the left lateral ventricle that is isointense to gray matter on T1 weighted images (black arrow). **B.** A more rostral axial T1 weighted image also shows a gray matter heterotopia in a band like distribution (white arrow).

Clinical-Radiological Diagnosis: Gray matter heterotopia.

KEY FACTS

Neuronal migrational abnormalities that can be a cause of seizures include schizencephaly (An abnormal gray matter lined cleft extending from a ventricle to the cortical surface), the pachygyria/polymicrogyria complex, and grey matter heterotopias. Gray matter heterotopias are divided into subependymal, subcortical, and band heterotopias. Band heterotopias present earlier than nodular (subependymal and subcortical) heterotopias, with developmental delay, and more severe seizure episodes.

REFERENCE

Barkovich AJ, Kuzniecky RI. Grey matter heterotopia. *Neurology.* 2000;55:1603–8.

CASE 10-3

A 6-year-old child is affected by medically-refractory seizures. Three types of seizures have been recognized: (1) generalized tonic-clonic seizures, (2) absence seizures, and (3) gelastic seizures (spontaneous laughing). Aside from seizures, this child shows signs of mild mental retardation and precocious puberty.

Neuroimaging is shown in Figs. 10-3-1 to 10-3-2.

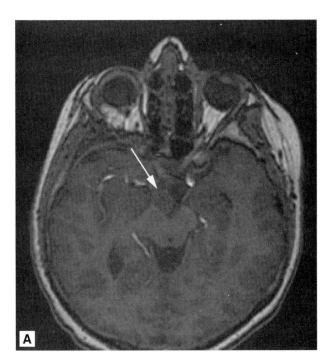

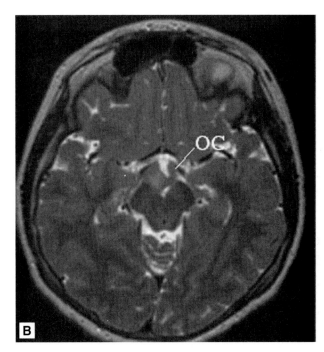

FIG. 10-3-1 **A.** Axial T1 and **B.** T2 MRIs. These images are remarkable for the presence of a homogeneous rounded lesion located between the optic chiasm and the right cerebral peduncle. On post-contrast T1, the lesion (arrrow) displays mild hyperintensity compared to brain parenchyma and does not contrast enhance. On T2, the lesion appears as a hyperintense mass adjacent to the optic chiasm (OC).

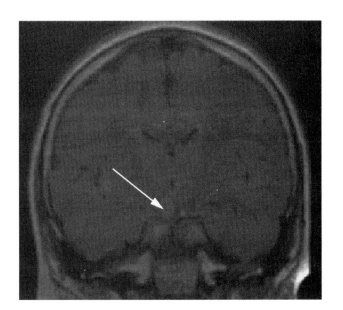

FIG. 10-3-2 Coronal T1. The white arrow points to the lesion which is clearly originating from the right hypothalamus. Again, mild hyperintensity is present.

Clinical-Radiological Diagnosis: Hypothalamic hamartoma.

KEY FACTS

Hypothalamic hamartomas are rare lesions typically associated with gelastic seizures. Mental retardation and precocious puberty can be variably associated. Recordings using depth electrodes have demostrated that this is an epileptogenic lesion. Surgical or radiosurgical ablation of hypothalamic hamartomas is associated with seizure regression.

CASE 10-4

A 38-year-old woman had several prolonged febrile seizures as a young child. She was treated with phenobarbital for 2 years and then developed normally and was seizure free until age 28. At that time, she began having olfactory hallucinations. Within 1 year, she went on to have complex partial seizures, occasionally with secondary generalization. They have been difficult to control with medications. Video EEG has identified a right temporal onset for most of her seizures.

Neuroimaging is shown in Figs. 10-4-1–10-4-2.

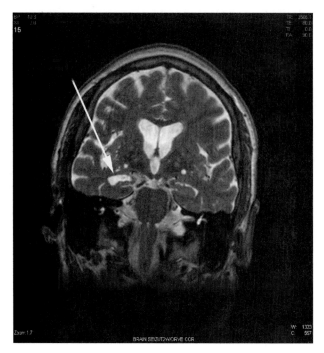

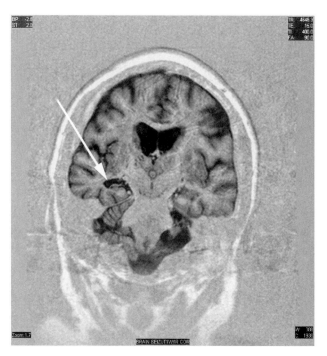

FIG. 10-4-1 T2 weighted MRI. This image demonstrates an abnormality in the right mesial temporal lobe. It is shrunken and malformed with enlargement of the temporal horn of the lateral ventricle. There is also a small area of abnormal high T2 signal within the right hippocampus. The left hippocampus is relatively normal.

Clinical-Radiological Diagnosis: Mesial temporal sclerosis.

FIG. 10-4-2 The T1 weighted image demonstrates the lesion with somewhat better anatomical detail.

KEY FACTS

Mesial temporal sclerosis is radiologically characterized by high T2 signal and loss of normal size and morphology. It is the most common cause of epilepsy in adults.

Chapter 11

BRAIN GENETIC DISORDERS

CASE 11-1

The patient is a 4-year-old boy with seizures, developmental delay, and increased head circumference.

Neuroimaging is shown in Figs. 11-1-1–11-1-7.

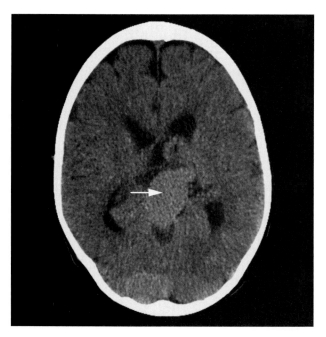

FIG. 11-1-1 Initial Head CT shows an abnormally enlarged midline draining vein (white arrow).

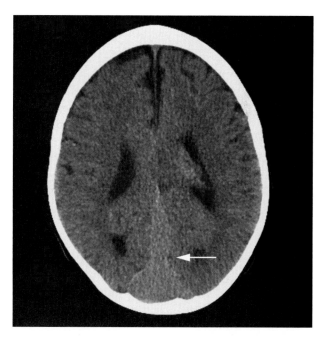

FIG. 11-1-2 This abnormal venous structure is in direct contiguity with the torcula (white arrow).

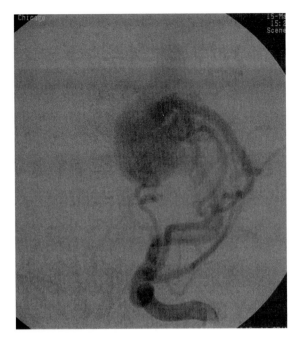

FIG. 11-1-3 Initial angiogram of the left internal carotid artery shows a large vein of Galen malformation fed by branches of the left middle cerebral artery as well as choroidal branches of the posterior cerebral arteries.

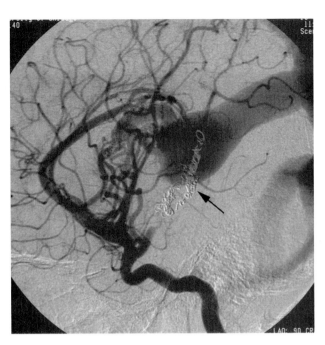

FIG. 11-1-5 Lateral angiogram nicely demonstrates successful emboliztion of multiple choroidal feeders (black arrow).

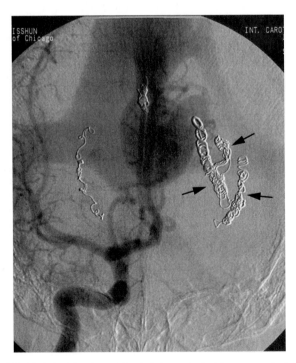

FIG. 11-1-4 The size of the draining vein in this case precluded coil placement in the vein of Galen itself from either an arterial or venous femoral approach. Multiple arterial feeders were embolized to reduce the flow. The coils are in choroidal branches of the posterior cerebral arteries bilaterally that supplied this malformation (black arrows).

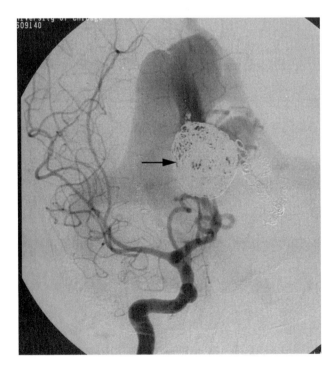

FIG. 11-1-6 The malformation was then embolized from a direct torcular approach. A large coil mass is seen in the draining vein (black arrow).

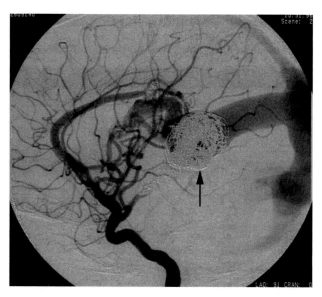

FIG. 11-1-7 Lateral angiogram again shows the large coil mass within the vein of Galen malformation, with reduced flow in the malformation (black arrow).

Clinical-Radiological Diagnosis: Vein of Galen malformation.

KEY FACTS

Normally the vein of Galen connects the deep venous drainage system (internal cerebral veins and basal veins of Rosenthal) to the straight sinus. In a vein of Galen malformation, the actual dilated vein is the primitive median prosencephalic vein of Markowski. The primary arterial supply to these lesions is usually from posterior choroidal branches and anterior cerebral artery branches. These lesions may present in infancy with high output cardiac failure or later in life with hydrocephalus, developmental delay, and failure to thrive, or hemorrhage. Primary treatment of these lesions is through endovascular means, by arterial or venous femoral approaches, though in difficult cases they may be approached through a direct venous approach.

REFERENCES

Horowitz MB, Jungreis CA, Quisling RG, Pollack I. Vein of Galen Aneurysms: a review and current perspective. *Prog Neurol Surg.* 2005;17:216–31.

Lasjuanias P, Garcia-Monaco R, Rodesch G, et al. Vein of Galen malformation. Endovascular management of 43 cases. *Child Nerv Syst.* 1991;7(7):360–7.

CASE 11-2

The patient is a 9-year-old girl with a long-standing history of seizures, mild mental retardation, a decreased attention span, as well as a pink papillary lesion in a malar distribution.

Neuroimaging is shown in Figs. 11-2-1–11-2-6.

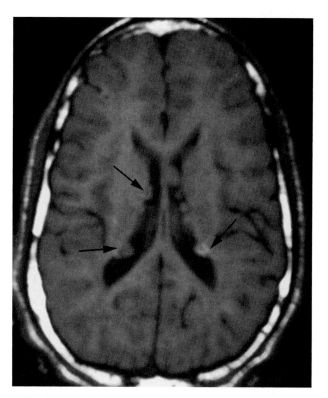

FIG. 11-2-1 Axial T1 weighted image shows multiple subependymal nodules that are isointense to gray matter lining both lateral ventricles (black arrows).

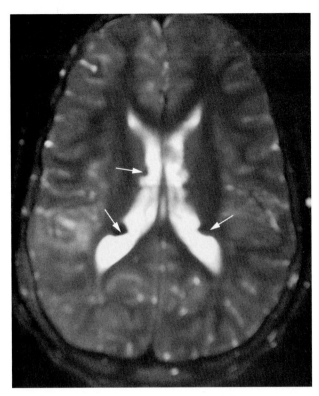

FIG. 11-2-2 Axial T2 weighted image confirms the presence of multiple low signal nodules lining the walls of the lateral ventricles (white arrows).

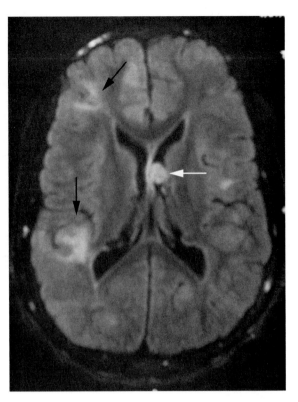

FIG. 11-2-4 Axial FLAIR image shows the mass lesion in the left lateral ventricle at the junction with the foramen of Munro to be of high signal intensity (white arrow). In addition there are multiple areas of high signal in the white matter (black arrows).

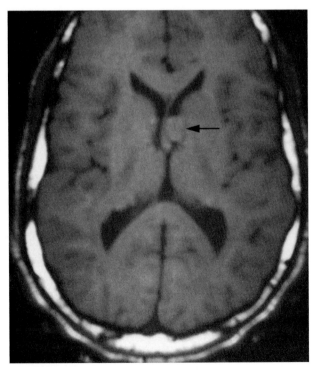

FIG. 11-2-3 Axial precontrast T1 weighted image shows a mass lesion in the left lateral ventricle at the foramen of Munro on the left (black arrow).

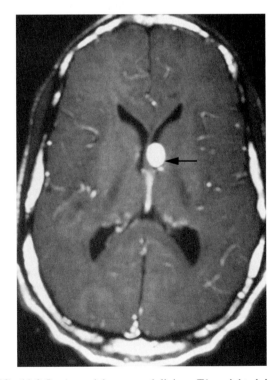

FIG. 11-2-5 An axial post gadolinium T1 weighted image shows the nodule in the left foramen of Munro to enhance homogenously (black arrow).

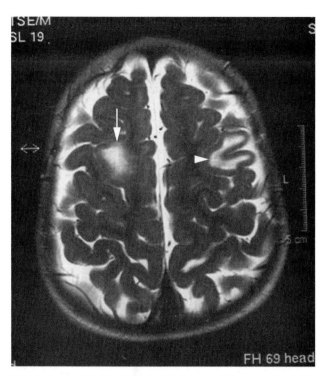

FIG. 11-2-6 A T2 weighted MRI from a different patient with the same condition showing a superior right frontal gyrus (white arrow) and a middle left frontal gyrus (white arrowhead) nodule. The cortical surface of these hyperintense nodules is lined by a layer of gray matter.

Clinical-Radiological Diagnosis: Tuberous sclerosis.

KEY FACTS

Tuberous sclerosis is a multisystem autosomal dominant disorder, which classically is characterized by a clinical triad of mental retardation, seizures, and adenoma sebaceum. The diagnostic criteria include two major features or one major and two minor features. The major features for this disorder are facial angiofibromas, hypomelanotic nodules, shagreen patch, cortical tuber, subependymal nodule, subependymal giant cell astrocytoma, retinal hamartomas, cardiac rhabdomyomas, lymphangioleiomyomatosis, and renal angiomyolipomas. Minor features include hamartomatous rectal polyps, dental pits, bone cysts, gingival fibromas, non-renal hamartomas, retinal achromic patch, "confetti" skin lesions, and multiple renal cysts.

Classic imaging findings in the central nervous system include cortical tubers, which are seen as high T2 signal intensity lesions in the white matter, subependymal nodules, which are often calcified, and can enhance. Subependymal giant cell astrocytomas characteristically arise in the region of the foramen of Munro and show homogenous enhancement.

REFERENCES

Barkovich AJ. Pediatric Neuroimaging. Philadelphia, PA: Lippincott, Williams, and Wilkins. 2005:556–7.

Curatolo P, Verdecchia M, Bombardieri R. Tuberous Sclerosis Complex: a Review of Neurologic Aspects. *Eur J Pediatr Neurol.* 2002;6:15–23.

Weiner DM, Ewalt DH, Roach ES, Hensle TW. The Tuberous sclerosis complex: A Comprehensive Review. *J Am Coll Surg.* 1998;187(5):548–561.

Wippold FJ, Baber WW, Gado M, Tobben PJ, Bartnicke BJ. Pre- and postcontrast MR studies in tuberous sclerosis. *J Comput Assist Tomogr.* 1992;16(1):69–72.

CASE 11-3

A 34-year-old man is evaluated for pain and weakness in the lower extremities. His previous medical history is remarkable for resection of an intracranial tumor 7 years ago. The patient reports that the tumor resection was complicated by severe bleeding originating from the tumor itself. Other intracranial lesions have developed over the years. Some relatives share a similar problem. Spastic paraparesis is detected following neurological exam. Fundoscopic examination reveals the presence of retinal angiomas.

Neuroimaging is shown in Fig. 11-3-1.

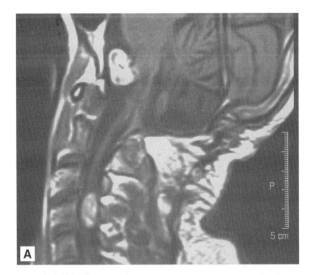

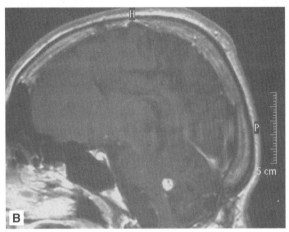

FIG. 11-3-1   A. Sagittal postcontrast T1 weighted brain and spinal MR show two homogeneously enhancing lesions on the same cut, one in the posterior fossa anterior to the bulb and the other at C4 level lateral to the spinal cord. **B.** A midline cut shows a third lesion located in the fourth ventricle. These lesions grow outside the brain and spinal cord and display a bright enhancement with some small non-enhancing areas. Brain and spinal cord appear atrophic.

Clinical-Radiological Diagnosis: Von Hippel-Lindau disease.

KEY FACTS

This is a genetic disorder causing the development of multiple hemangioblastomas. The CNS is a common location with multiple intracranial and spinal lesions easily detected on neuroimaging. Hemangioblastomas are the most common posterior cranial fossa tumors in adults. Other phakomatoses such as NF1 and NF2 can be differentiated on the basis of the history of severe intraoperative bleeding and the marked contrast enhancement (suggesting vascular lesions) while neurofibromas and schwannomas are characterized by modest or poor enhancement.

CASE 11-4

The patient is a 3-month-old girl with nausea, vomiting, irritability, and a tense fontanelle on physical examination. Neuroimaging is shown in Figs. 11-4-1–11-4-2.

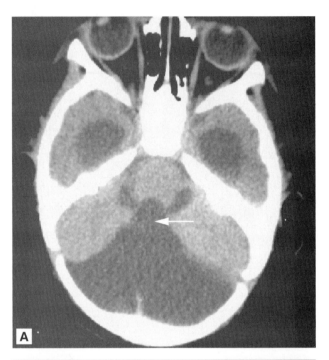

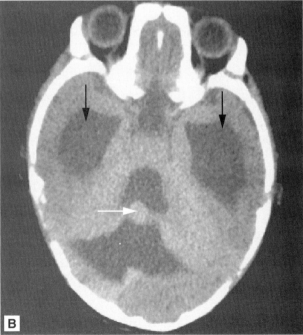

FIG. 11-4-1   A. Noncontrast head CT shows a communication between an enlarged cystic dilatation of the posterior fossa and the fourth ventricle with a classic "keyhole" appearance (white arrow). **B.** The superior portion of the vermis is present (white arrow). There is marked dilatation of the temporal horns of the lateral ventricles (black arrows).

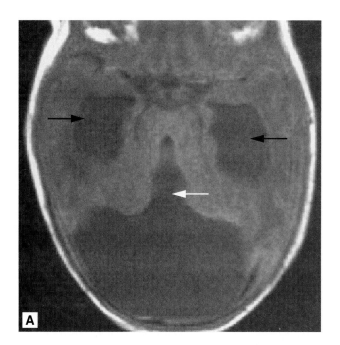
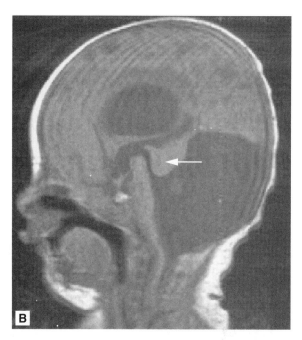

FIG. 11-4-2   A. Left and Right: MRI scan from a different patient also shows a large posterior fossa cyst on pre-contrast T1 weighted images with a connection to the 4th ventricle (white arrow). There is hydrocephalus with dilatation of the temporal horns of both ventricles (black arrows). **B.** On sagittal T1 weighted images there is partial vermian agenesis (the white arrow demonstrates the remnant vermis).

Clinical-Radiological Diagnosis: Dandy Walker variant malformation.

KEY FACTS

A Dandy Walker malformation has complete vermian agenesis, while a Dandy Walker variant has only partial vermian agenesis.

CASE 11-5

The patient is a 21-year-old woman with a history of cerebral palsy and seizures, now with an increase in seizure frequency.

Neuroimaging is shown in Figs. 11-5-1–11-5-3.

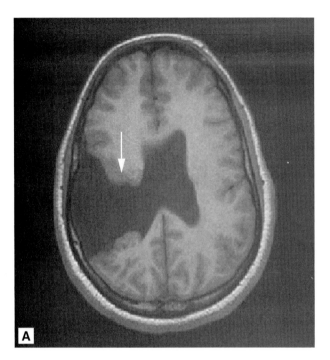

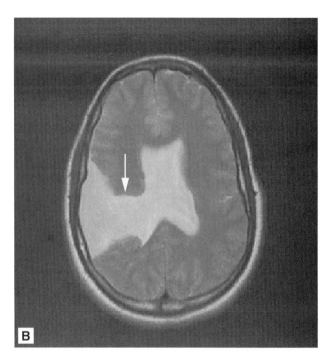

FIG. 11-5-1 **A.** Axial T1 weighted MRI image shows a gray matter lined cleft extending from the right lateral ventricle to the pial cortical surface (white arrow). **B.** This is also seen on axial T2 weighted images. Notice the large gap (filled with CSF) between the gray matter lining of the cleft (white arrow).

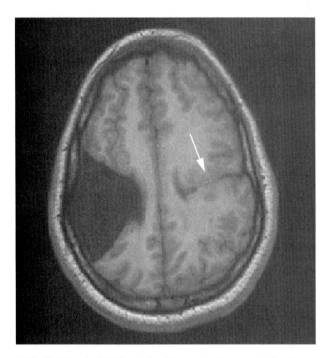

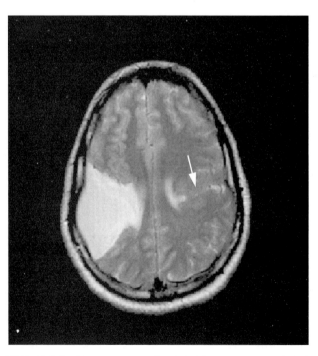

FIG. 11-5-2 Axial T1 weighted image (white arrow) also shows a gray matter lined CSF cleft on the left side extending from the left lateral ventricle to the pial covering of the cortex. The gray matter clefts are more closely apposed on the left.

FIG. 11-5-3 The gray matter lined cleft is also seen on axial T2 weighted images (white arrow).

Clinical-Radiological Diagnosis: Open lipped schizencephaly on the right. Closed lipped schizencephaly on left.

KEY FACTS

Schizencephaly is a migrational abnormality characterized by the presence of a gray matter lined cleft extending from a ventricle to the cortical surface. There are closed (gray matter lining closely apposed) and open lipped (separation of gray matter lining) varieties. Patients with bilateral defects tend to have more severe developmental delay and seizures than patients with unilateral clefts. Associated abnormalities can include midline hypoplasias of the optic tracts or pituitary, as well as absence of the septum pellucidum or partial agenesis of the corpus callosum.

REFERENCE

Barkovich AJ, Kjos BO. Schizencephaly: correlation of clinical findings with MR characteristics. *Am J Neuroradiol.* 1992;13(1):85–94.

CASE 11-6

A 2-year-old girl who was conceived by first degree cousins is evaluated for psychomotor delay and myoclonic seizures. Over time, progressive neurological and cognitive deterioration has developed. EEG shows diffuse, severe slowing and frequent, generalized spike and waves. Cutaneous biopsy is then performed indicating a diagnosis of Ceroid lipofuscinosis type II (Jansky-Bielschowsky type). Loss of vision at 5 years is followed by exitus at age 7.

Neuroimaging is shown in Figs. 11-6-1–11-6-2.

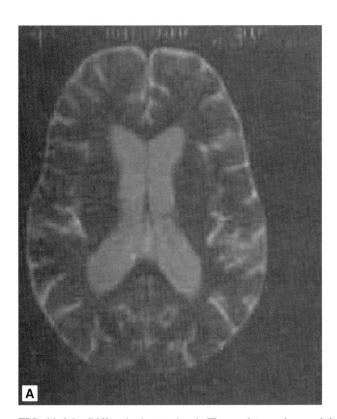
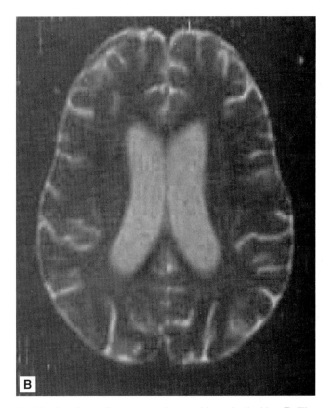

FIG. 11-6-1 Diffuse brain atrophy. **A.** The caudate nucleus and the rest of the basal ganglia are severely atrophic on both sides. **B.** The lateral ventricles are enlarged due to the atrophy of the hemispheric white matter. Cortical sulci are diffusely widened in both images.

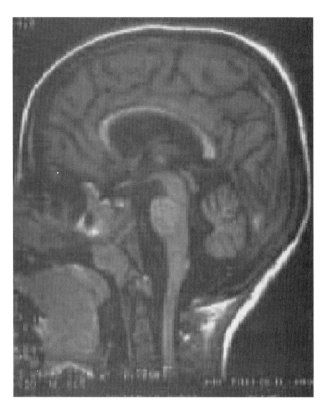

FIG. 11-6-2 Sagittal T1 MRI also shows diffuse atrophy, involving the corpus callosum, the cortex, and the cerebellum.

Clinical-Radiological Diagnosis: Inherited metabolic disorder (ceroid lipofuscinosis)

KEY FACTS

Late infantile (Jansky-Bielschowsky) is the most common type of neuronal ceroid lipofuscinosis. The presentation begins with myoclonic seizures between ages 2–4 years. The clinical course includes dementia, ataxia, progressive visual loss, and microcephaly.

CASE 11-7

An 18-month-old girl with severe psychomotor delay develops myoclonic spasms. Pregnancy was characterized by early termination with C-section at 7 months because of preeclampsia. Weight at birth was 1.2 kg. Apgar score was 5. A diagnosis of West syndrome is made on the basis of the seizure semiology and pattern plus EEG showing diffuse epileptogenic activity, mostly originating from right hemisphere, superimposed on a slow and poorly organized background. Neurological exam is remarkable for spastic diplegia.

Neuroimaging is shown in Fig. 11-7-1.

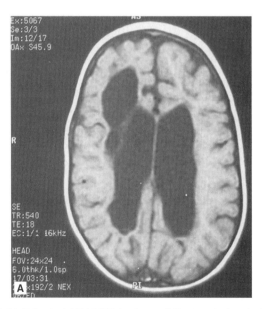
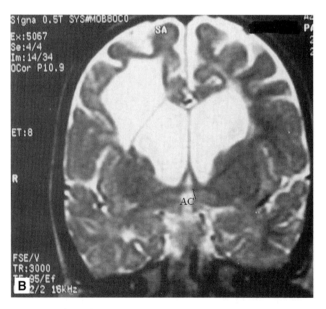

FIG. 11-7-1 Axial T1 MRI **A.** shows diffuse cortical and white matter atrophy, enlarged lateral ventricles and a large porencephalic cyst located in the right frontal lobe. On coronal T2 **B,** a tiny septum dividing the right ventricle from the cyst can be appreciated. Signal intensity of the cyst content is the same as CSF on both sequences (hypointense in T1, hyperintense on T2). The coronal cut shows the near total absence of hemispheric white matter while the anterior commissure (AC) is grossly normal.

Clinical-Radiological Diagnosis: Periventricular leucomalacia with porencephalic cyst.

KEY FACTS

West syndrome is a severe seizure disorder of infancy, which may be due to any of a number of causes of perinatal brain damage.

REFERENCE

Raffaella Cusmai, Stefano Ricci, Jean Marc Pinard et al. West syndrome due to perinatal insults. *Epilepsia.* 1993;34(4): 73&742.

CASE 11-8

A 16-year-old girl is referred to a pain specialist because she is affected by left-sided facial pain involving the territory of the second and third branch of the trigeminal nerve. The pain is dull and constant. A steady worsening has been noticed over the last year. The parents report that she was recently diagnosed with a bone disease affecting the skull base and causing stenosis of the left optic canal with consequent visual failure. A cranioplasty was performed in order to relieve the pressure exerted on the optic apparatus and the consequent visual failure. The craniotomy was followed by full visual recovery.

Neuroimaging is shown in Figs. 11-8-1–11-8-5. Following injection of IV contrast, no uptake occurs (not shown).

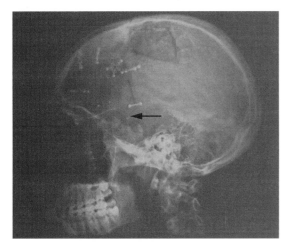

FIG. 11-8-1 Skull plain x-ray (lateral view). An orbito-frontal bone flap with metallic fixation devices is evident. This surgical approach was used to expose and decompress the optic nerve within the optic canal. Remodelling of the orbital vault was achieved using a titanium mesh (black arrow). Focal homogenous thickening of the occipital bone can be appreciated.

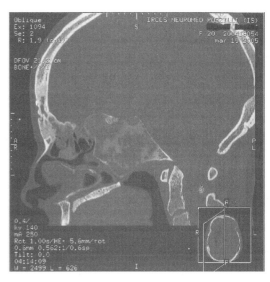

FIG. 11-8-2 Head CT illustrates a sagittal midline cut using a bone window. The sphenoid and ethmoid bones are grossly thickened. In the sphenoid bone, predominant cystic areas are intermixed with islands of dysplastic diploic bone. The sphenoid sinus is nearly obliterated by the dysplastic tissue. The ethmoid bone is also thickened while the cranial vault shows regions of focal bony sclerosis or diploic thickening.

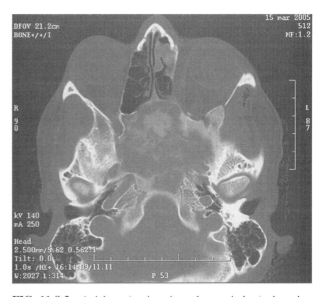

FIG. 11-8-3 Axial cut (again using a bone window): the sphenoid bone is quite enlarged and deformed by the dysplastic tissue. This tissue displays homogenous signal with a density less than normal bone. Several cystic regions are clearly appreciated. The dysplastic growth is asymmetric, with a larger involvement of the bony structures on the left side, suggesting an encroachment of the trigeminal branches. Higher cuts (not illustrated) show that there is no bony encroachment over the left Meckel's cave.

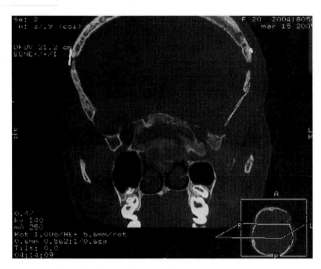

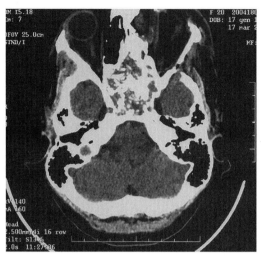

FIG. 11-8-4   A coronal cut through the sphenoid bone, showing the dysplastic tissue bordered superiorly by sclerotic bone. The cranioplasty site is indicated by the mesh, clearly visible on the right side (patient's left side) as a bright lucency with regular, circular holes.

FIG. 11-8-5   An axial cut using a brain window. The dysplastic tissue appears as a dyshomogenous mass with an irregular mix of hyperdensity and hypodensity related, respectively, to areas of calcified bone and of fibrous tissue.

Clinical-Radiological Diagnosis: Fibrous dysplasia of the skull.

KEY FACTS

Fibrous dysplasia is a benign disorder of the bone characterized by the replacement of normal bone with highly vascular fibro-osseous connective tissue. Three radiological varieties can be identified: cystic (focal homogenous widening of the diploes, more commonly affecting the cranial vault), sclerotic (diffuse skull base thickening, especially affecting the sphenoid bone), and mixed. Cranial nerve foramina are usually preserved but in some cases surgical decompression may be required. The disease is active mostly during adolescence becoming stable when the adulthood is reached. Fibrous dysplasia is usually a focal process and, on this basis, can be easily distinguished from Paget's disease, characterized by systemic symptoms and diffuse thickening of the skull with distorted trabecular pattern.

Chapter 12

DEGENERATIVE DISEASE AND DEMENTIA

CASE 12-1

A 48-year-old man carries the diagnosis of juvenile onset Parkinson's disease. This disease was diagnosed 8 years ago on the basis of the progressive development of resting tremor, bradykinesia and rigidity on the left side equally affecting arm and leg and then crossing to the opposite side. Optimal response to dopaminergic medications was experienced by this patient for over 5 years, followed by the development of the typical complications induced by long-term administration of such drugs (dyskinesias, associated with on-off phenomena and freezing). Following evaluation by a multidisciplinary team, including a neurologist specialized in movement disorders, a functional neurosurgeon, and a dedicated neuropsychologist, he was offered the option of implanting a subthalamic nucleus (STN) deep brain stimulation device (DBS) bilaterally in order to optimize the symptomatic control of the disease and to reduce the administration of dopaminergic drugs, with consequent reduction of drug-related symptoms. A DBS was placed without complications in the right STN. Microelectrode recording confirmed the DBS placement in the STN sensorimotor region. Excellent microlesion effect was detected after the DBS implantation with near total contralateral resolution of rigidity and tremor. Dopaminergic drugs could be substantially reduced and dyskinesias disappeared. After 6 weeks, a

brain MRI is performed to direct the targeting of the contralateral DBS.

Neuroimaging is shown in Figs. 12-1-1–12-1-3.

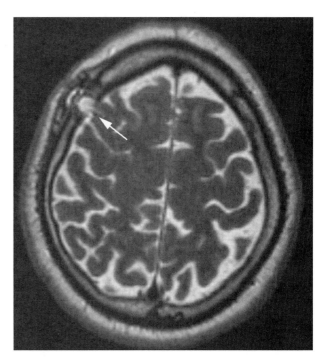

FIG. 12-1-1 Axial T2 MRI cut at the level of the burr hole. The DBS penetrating the cortex through the second frontal gyrus is visible immediately below the burr hole as a small hyperintense signal (white arrow). A modest degree of brain atrophy can be appreciated by the wide size of the sulci.

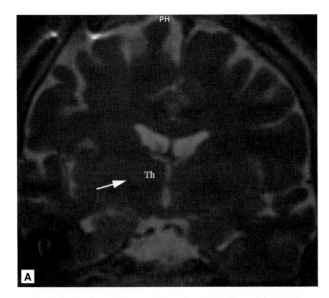

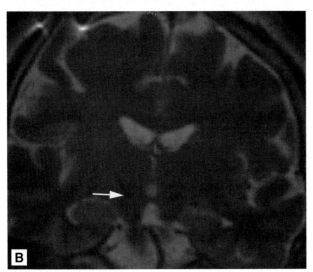

FIG. 12-1-2 A coronal T2 MRI is very useful to follow the DBS pathway through brain. Typically, a DBS directed to the STN penetrates the frontal lobe anteriorly to the sensorimotor cortex, coming through the corona radiata, the outer shell of the thalamus (reticular thalamus), the zona incerta (a white matter region between the ventral border of the thalamus and the STN), and finally the STN itself. DBS electrodes provide 4 contacts: the deeper contact is usually placed immediately below the STN in the pars reticulata of the substantia nigra, two intermediate contacts are placed within the STN and the upper contact in the zona incerta. Microelectrode recording helps to identify these structures before the final DBS implantation. **A.** Shows the DBS as an elongated hypointense signal (arrow) along the lateral border of the thalamus (Th). **B.** Shows the tip of the DBS in the subthalamic region.

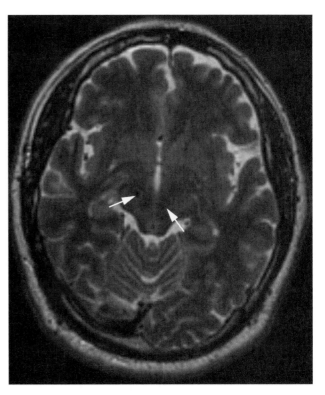

FIG. 12-1-3 Axial T2 MRI performed using thin cuts (2 mm) shows the tip of the DBS placed lateral and anterior to the red nucleus. A fast spin-echo (FSE) sequence is typically used for stereotactic localization. The arrow on the patient's right shows a markedly hypointense circular signal surrounded by a thin hyperintense halo, which is the typical DBS appearance on T2 weighted imaging. The hyperintense halo is likely related to local edema and may disappear over time. The arrow on the left points to the contour of the red nucleus, a precious landmark for the surgeon targeting the subthalamic nucleus, due to a quite reliable spatial relationship with the subthalamic nucleus, which is in most cases a few millimetres lateral to the anterior border of the red nucleus.

Clinical-Radiological Diagnosis: Right STN DBS placement.

KEY FACTS

Some brain atrophy is a common finding in patients with Parkinson's disease. The ability to reliably identify the red nucleus (which is easily visualized as a rounded slightly hypointense structure in the upper brainstem close to the midline) and the STN (this nucleus is slightly anterior, superior, and lateral to the red nucleus and does not display clear borders) is the reason why stereotactic procedures base STN localization on FSE T2 sequences.

Chapter 13

BENIGN MRI AND CT FINDINGS

CASE 13-1

A 21-year-old normally developed healthy man was walking toward his car in the parking lot after shopping. The next thing that he remembers is being tied down to a backboard by paramedics. Witnesses had seen a generalized tonic clonic seizure lasting approximately 1 minute, followed by confusion. There were no semiological features to suggest a focal onset. EEG showed frequent bursts of 5–6 Hz generalized spike-wave and polyspikes.

Neuroimaging is shown in Fig. 13-1-1.

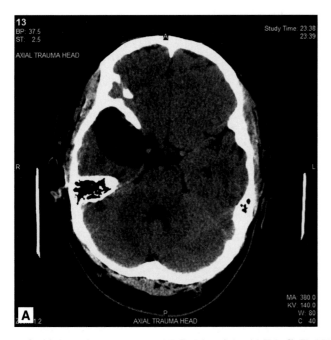 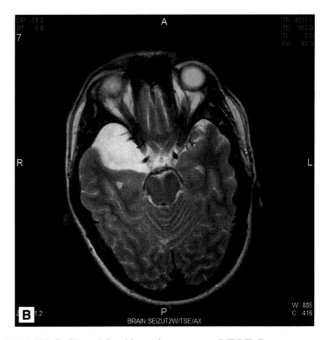

FIG. 13-1-1 A. Noncontrast CT. **B.** T2 weighted MRI. **C.** FLAIR (T2) MRI. **D.** T1 weighted inversion recovery MRI **E.** Postcontrast T1 MRI. The images show a mass located within the middle cranial fossa. It is noncalcified with imaging characteristics similar to CSF on CT and all MRI sequences. There is no enhancement following contrast administration. *(Continued)*

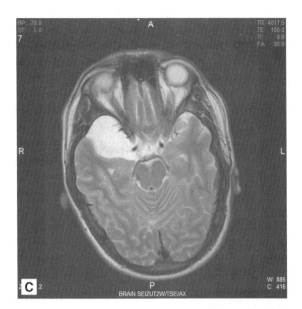

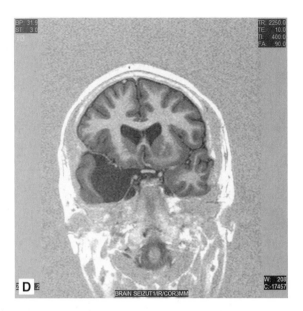

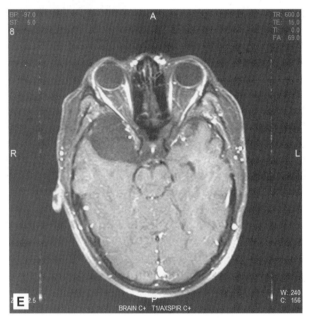

FIG. 13-1-1 *(Continued)*

Clinical-Radiological Diagnosis: Arachnoid cyst. Arachnoid cysts have occasionally been implicated as a cause of seizures, but in this case it appears to be an incidental finding in a patient with newly diagnosed primary generalized epilepsy.

KEY FACTS

An arachnoid cyst is a congenital extra-axial cerebrospinal fluid containing mass (caused by splitting of the arachnoid). On imaging, these cysts follow CSF on all imaging modalities. They are usually asymptomatic, but can rarely cause seizures or headaches.

CASE 13-2

An 18-year-old woman had an MRI ordered by her primary care doctor because of frontal-temporal throbbing headaches. She has been sent to see a neurologist because of a possible abnormality on her MRI. The headaches are consistent with typical common migraine.

Neuroimaging is shown in Figs. 13-2-1 to 13-2-2.

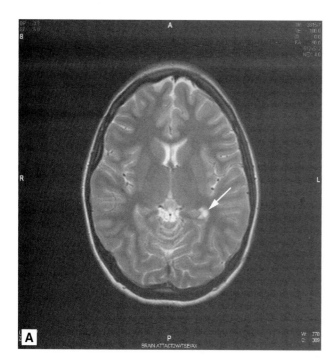
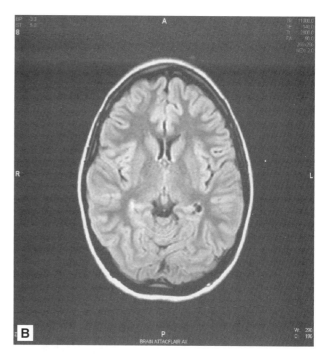

FIG. 13-2-1   A. T2 TSE. **B.** T2 FLAIR images demonstrating the suspected lesion. The finding is located within the trigone of the left lateral ventricle.

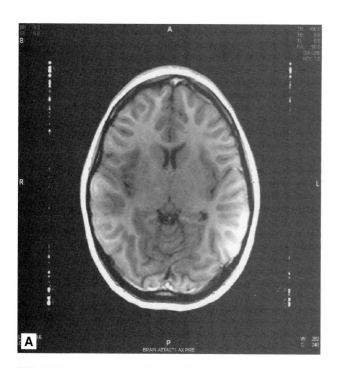
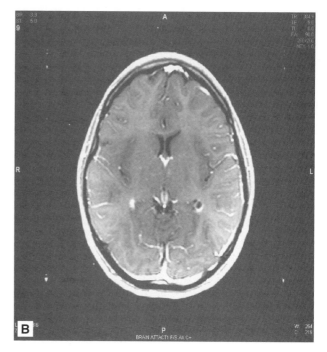

FIG. 13-2-2   A. Pre- and **B.** Post-Contrast T1 weighted images further confirm that the structure in question has signal characteristics similar to CSF. The enhancement around the cystic structure is the glomus of the choroid plexus.

Clinical-Radiological Diagnosis: Choroid plexus cyst.

KEY FACTS

Choroid plexus cysts are non-neoplastic epithelial lined cysts of no known clinical significance. They are often bilateral and have signal characteristics generally similar to CSF. Approximately 1% of patients have a "cyst-like" appearance of the glomus of the choroid plexus. DWI most often shows high signal in at least part of the cyst, but may not.

REFERENCES

Kinoshita T, Moritani T, Hiwatashi A et al. T. Clinically silent choroid plexus cyst: evaluation by diffusion-weighted MRI. *Neuroradiology.* 2005 Apr;47(4):251–5.

Koopmans RA, Li DK, Paty DW. Glomus of the choroid plexus: the normal spin-echo appearance on magnetic resonance imaging. *Can Assoc Radiol J.* 1990 Aug;41(4):195–200.

CASE 13-3

A 50-year-old woman with a many year history of partial onset seizures and mental illness.

Neuroimaging is shown in Fig. 13-3-1.

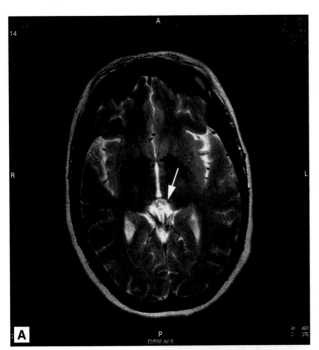

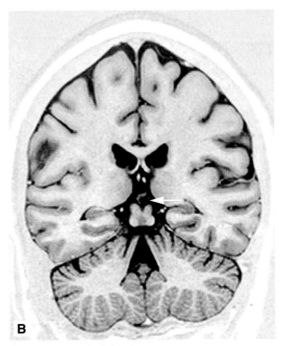

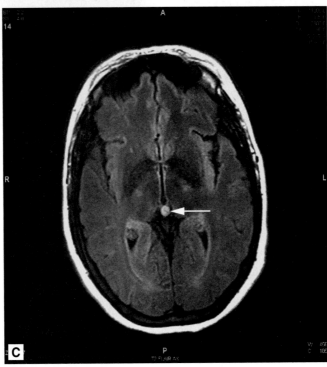

FIG. 13-3-1   A. T2 **B.** T1 with inversion recovery **C.** FLAIR. The above images show a small pineal mass which has a relatively smooth margin and contains material with high T2 signal (white arrow).

Clinical-Radiological Diagnosis: Benign pineal cyst.

KEY FACTS

Pineal masses cannot be definitively diagnosed by MRI. However, a small smoothly marginated cystic lesion is suggestive of benign cysts which may be found in up to 40% of people at autopsy.

REFERENCE

Yukunori K, Mutsumasa T, Yukitaka U. MRI of pineal region tumors. *J Neurooncol.* 2001;54:251–61.

CASE 13-4

A 17-year-old woman had seen her primary care doctor because of headaches. They were posterior/occipital or left-sided, often accompanied by neck pain, occurring up 2–3 times per week. She described a constant throbbing or squeezing pain lasting for hours which was better with ibuprofen or lying down. Worse with light, noise, menstrual periods, or eating cold food. An MRI had been ordered and not followed up for 3 months. When the primary care doctor saw the MRI results, he immediately sent the patient to the emergency room for neurological evaluation. Neurological examination was normal.

Neuroimaging is shown in Figs. 13-4-1–13-4-2.

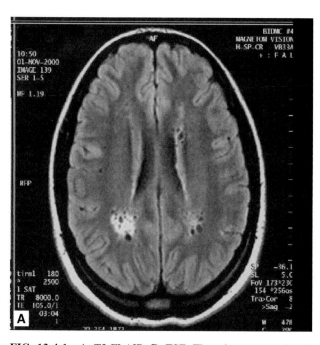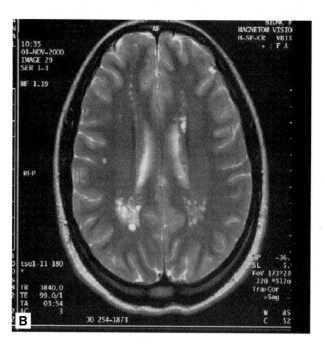

FIG. 13-4-1 A. T2 FLAIR. **B.** TSE. These images reveal multiple cyst-like or tubular structures within the white matter more in the posterior than anterior regions. There appears to be some associated high T2 signal within the white matter.

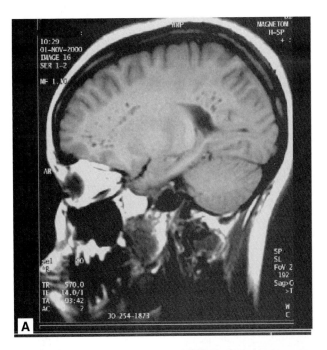
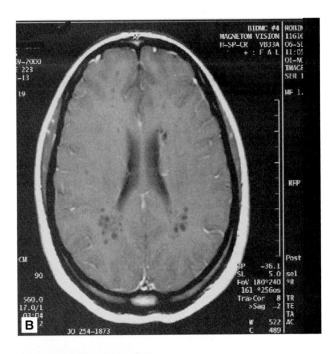

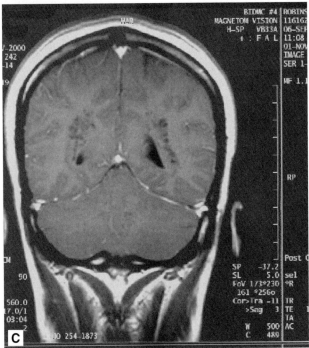

FIG. 13-4-2   A. Precontrast sagittal. **B and C.** Postcontrast axial and coronal T1 weighted images show that they are nonenhancing and converge toward the ventricles.

Clinical-Radiological Diagnosis: Prominent perivascular (Virchow-Robin) spaces. Incidental finding in patient with migraine/tension-type headaches.

pia mater and are a normal finding. All testing to exclude other diagnoses such as infections, vascular abnormality, or metabolic disease were negative in this case.

KEY FACTS

Virchow-Robin spaces are perivascular spaces surrounding the perforating arteries. They are extensions of the

REFERENCE

Eichhorn GR, Ammache Z, Bell W, Yuh WT. Unusually prominent perivascular spaces. *Neurology.* 2001 May 8;56(9):1242.

Chapter 14

VASCULAR LESIONS

CASE 14-1

A 45-year-old man with low back pain, and progressive lower extremity weakness over the past few months. In

the past few weeks he has developed bowel and bladder incontinence.

Neuroimaging is shown in Figs. 14-1-1–14-1-3.

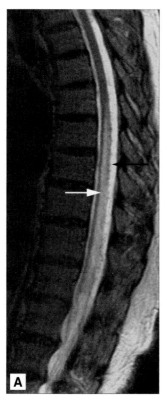
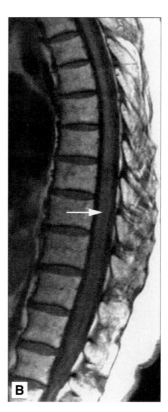
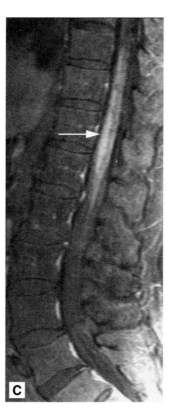

FIG. 14-1-1   A. T2 weighted image shows increased signal within in the lumbar spine (white arrow). Posteriorly there are abnormal flow voids on sagittal T2 weighted images (black arrow). **B.** Precontrast sagittal T1 weighted image shows low signal within the cord consistent with cord edema (white arrow). **C.** Postgadolinium T1 weighted image shows diffuse enhancement (white arrow). **D.** Axial T2 weighted images confirms high T2 signal in the cord. The differential diagnosis for the T2 signal abnormality and enhancement includes transverse myelitis, spinal cord infarct, and demyelinating disease. However, the presence of flow voids strongly suggests a vascular malformation as the cause. Tumors can cause T2 signal abnormality in the cord, but will usually show nodular enhancement within the cord, or leptomeningeal enhancement. *(Continued)*

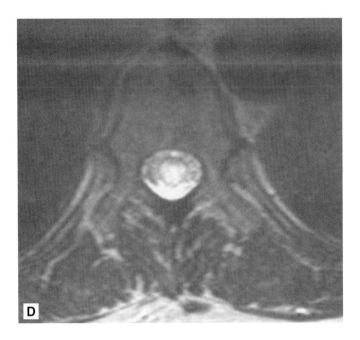

FIG. 14-1-1   *(Continued)*

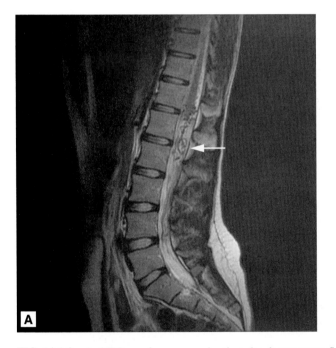

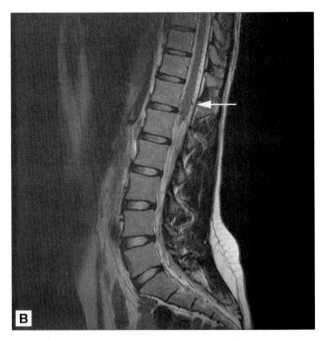

FIG. 14-1-2   An MRI scan from a second patient also demonstrates findings worrisome for a spine vascular malformation. There are abnormal serpiginous flow voids in a perimedullary location (white arrow) around the conus medullaris (A) as well as (B) along the posterior aspect of the cord, also marked by a white arrow.

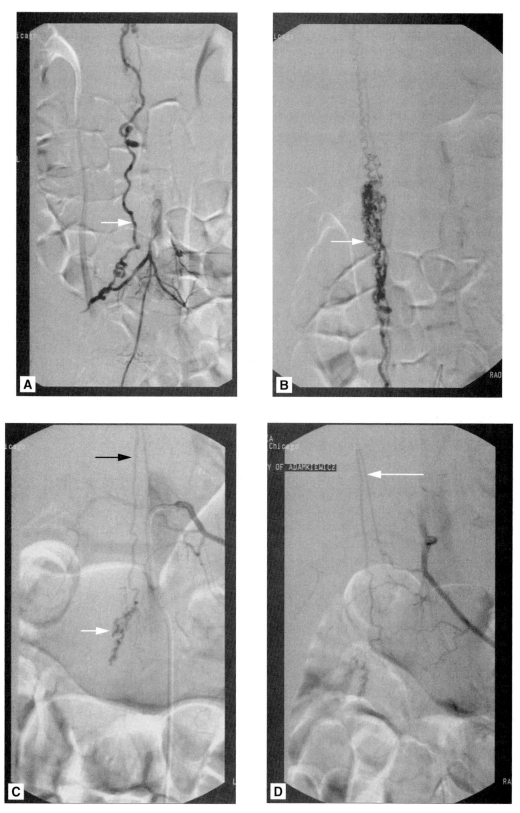

FIG. 14-1-3   **A.** Spinal angiography with selective injection of a branch supplying the median sacral artery as well as both L5 lumbar arteries shows a feeding vessel from the right L5 lumbar branch (white arrow) with two small aneurysms. **B.** Delayed images in the venous phase centered over the level of the conus medullaris shows a cranially draining venous plexus (white arrow). **C.** Selective injection of the left T 11 intercostal artery shows that there is supply to the nidus (white arrow) from the artery of Adamciewicz (black arrow) as well. **D.** Note the classic hairpin loop of the artery of Adamkiewicz (white arrow).

Clinical-Radiological Diagnosis: spinal arteriovenous malformation.

KEY FACTS

Spine vascular malformations are rare lesions that often present with a slowly progressive myelopathy. Early diagnosis is critical as this is a treatable cause of a progressive myelopathy. T2 signal abnormality, cord expansion, diffuse cord enhancement, and serpiginous flow voids are all signs of a spine vascular malformation. Spine angiograpy is the gold standard for diagnosis. The most common type of a spine vascular malformation is a dural arteriovenous fistula, or type 1 spine arteriovenous fistula (AVF). This is characterized by a single radicular branch feeding the lesion with an abnormal arteriovenous connection in a dural nerve sleeve, and presents with a slowly progressive myelopathy from venous hypertension. Type II and type III arteriovenous malformations (AVMs) have an intramedullary component, and can present with acute sudden neurologic deterioration. Type IV lesions are perimedullary fistulas usually supplied by the anterior spinal artery.

REFERENCE

Rodesch G, Lasjaunias P. Spinal cord arteriovenous shunts: from imaging to management. *Eur J Radiol.* 2003;46:221–32.

Chapter 15

SPINE TUMORS

CASE 15-1

A 31-year-old man with a history of Cafe Au Lait spots since childhood and axial/inguinal freckling. MRI done for routine follow up.

Neuroimaging is shown in Figs. 15-1-1–15-1-3.

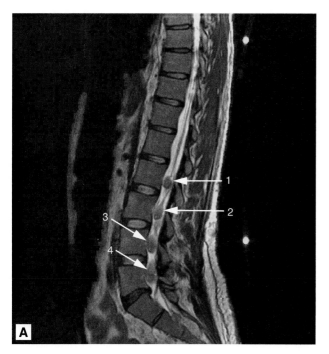
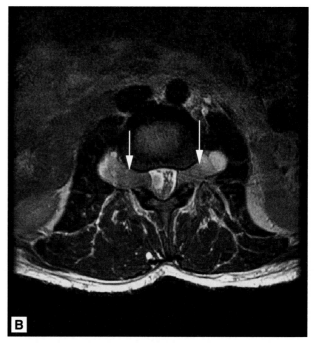

FIG. 15-1-1 **A.** Sagittal T2 weighted image shows an isointense mass in the expected location of the of the L2–L5 nerve roots on the left side (1–L2, 2–L3, 3–L4, 4–L5). **B.** Axial T2 weighted image shows bilateral L2 nerve root enlargement (white arrows).

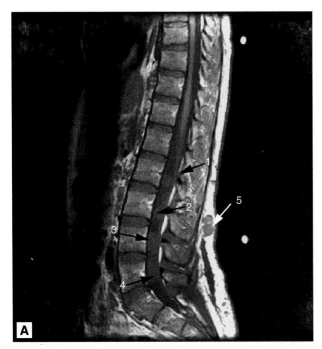
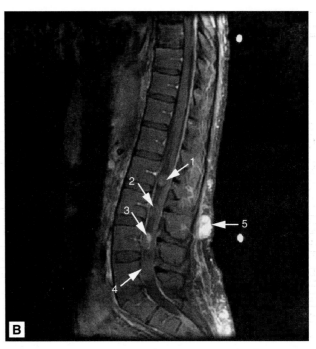

FIG. 15-1-2   A. Precontrast T1 weighted images again demonstrate isointense masses of the left L2 (1), L3 (2), L4 (3), and L5 (4) nerve roots. There is also a subcutaneous lesion (5) that is isointense on T1 weighted images to muscle. **B.** Post contrast T1 sagittal images show faint enhancement of the left L2 (1) and L3 (2) lesions, heterogenous enhancement of the left L4 lesion (3), and faint enhancement of the L5 (4) lesion. The subcutaneous nodule (5) enhances avidly.

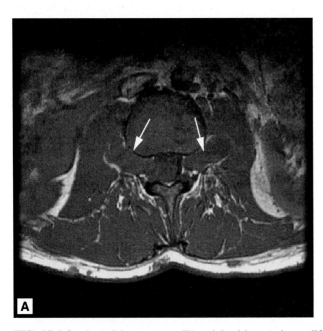
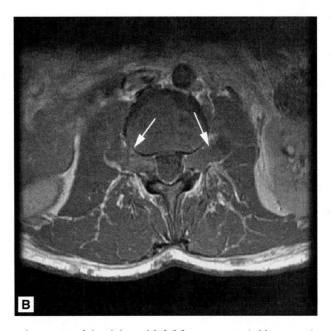

FIG. 15-1-3   A. Axial precontrast T1 weighted image shows diffuse enlargement of the right and left L2 nerve roots (white arrows), which show faint enhancement on **B.** post contrast T1 weighted images (white arrows).

Clincal-Radiologic Diagnosis: Neurofibromatosis Type 1.

KEY FACTS

Neurofibromatosis type 1, also known as Von Recklinghausen's disease is a neurocutaneous disorder with multiple systematic stigmata including Café au Lait skin lesions, plexiform neurofibromas, optic gliomas, iris hamartomas, sphenoid dysplasia, and pseudoarthroses of long bones. These patients also have characteristic high T2 signal lesions in gray matter. Plexiform neurofribromas can have malignant degeneration.

CASE 15-2

A 60-year-old man presented with 5 months of worsening dysesthesia radiating from the lower thoracic spine around to the rib cage. This was originally thought to have been from kidney stones.

Neuroimaging is shown in Figs. 15-2-1–15-2-4.

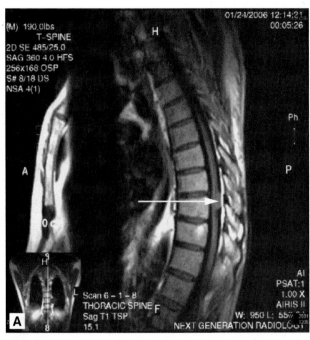
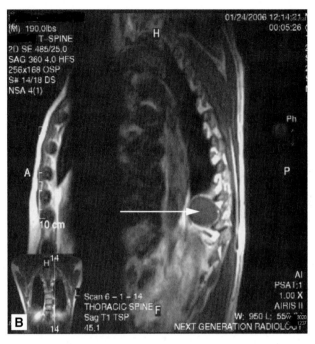

FIG. 15-2-1 Precontrast T1 weighted MRI reveals a low thoracic spine lesion with both intra **A.** and extra **B.** axial components.

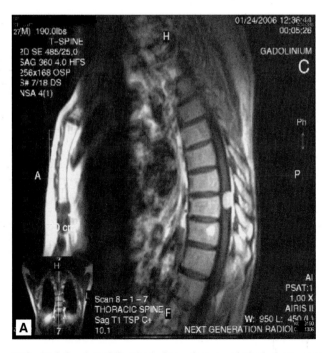
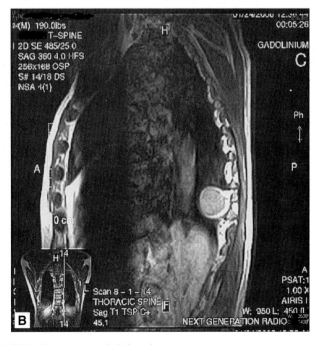

FIG. 15-2-2 **A and B.** The lesion enhances relatively homogenously following contrast administration.

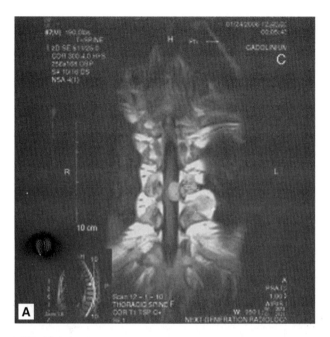

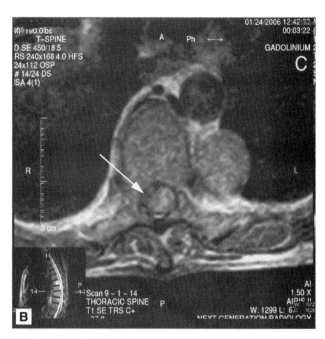

FIG. 15-2-3   A. The "dumbbell" morphology with a thin connecting bridge of tissue is more apparent on coronal and axial sequences (T1 postcontrast). **B.** The flattened spinal cord (white arrow) is easily visualized in the axial cut.

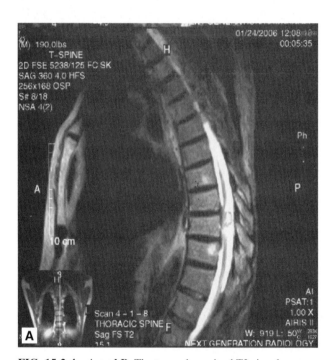

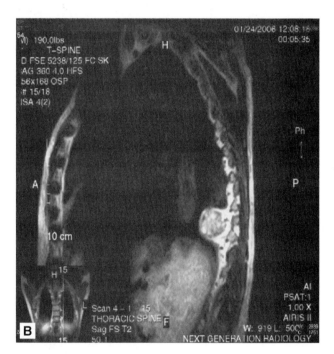

FIG. 15-2-4   A and B. The tumor has mixed T2 signal.

Clinical-Pathological-Radiological Diagnosis: Spindle cell neoplasm, probable schwannoma.

KEY FACTS

Schwannomas are the most common primary tumors of the spine. They are typically extramedullary with intra

and/or extradural components. Rarely an intramedullary component exists.

REFERENCE

Kono K, Inoue Y, Nakamura H, Shakudo M, Nakayama K. MR imaging of a case of a dumbbell-shaped spinal schwannoma with intramedullary and intradural-extramedullary components. *Neuroradiology.* 2001 Oct;43(10):864–7.

CASE 15-3

A 53-year-old woman with a history of neurofibromatosis and a recurrent spinal tumor presented to her surgeon with increasing right lower extremity pain and new left lower extremity pain. Her MRI showed slight worsening of her tumor compared with 6 months ago.

Neuroimaging is shown in Figs. 15-3-1–15-3-2.

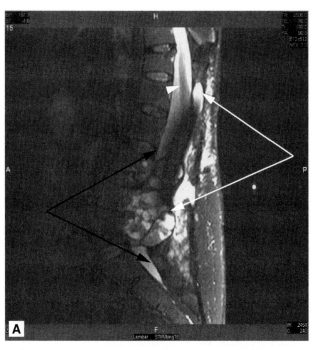
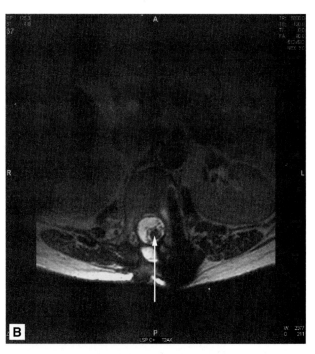

FIG. 15-3-1 **A.** Sagittal STIR/long TE sequence. Relevant findings include a susceptibility artifact due to previously implanted instrumentation (white arrows) and a massive heterogeneous paraspinal mass (black arrows). The spinal cord (arrowhead) within the canal may be seen rostral to the tumor. **B.** Axial T2 shows the conus medullaris (white arrow) surrounded by the start of the caude equina displaced toward the left.

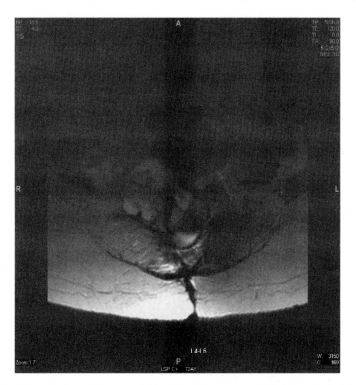

FIG. 15-3-2 At the L4–L5 level the spinal canal is completely effaced by tumor which has extended through the right neuroforamine and displaced the psoas muscle anteriorly.

Clinical-Pathological-Radiological Diagnosis: Cellular schwannoma with invasion of bone and soft tissue.

KEY FACTS

Schwannomas of the spine are generally benign and amenable to total resection; however, occasionally a malignant form occurs which carries a poorer prognosis.

REFERENCE

Conti P, Pansini G, Mouchaty H, Capuano C, Conti R. Spinal neurinomas: retrospective analysis and long-term outcome of 179 consecutively operated cases and review of the literature. *Surg Neurol.* 2004;61(1):34–43; discussion 44.

CASE 15-4

A 60-year-old man presented 10 years ago with gradually worsening weakness, worse in his lower extremities. He was found to have a cervical spine arachnoid cyst and treated by a midline myelotomy. He did well until within the past month he developed worsening paresthesias of his upper extremities and generalized weakness. Examination is significant for increased reflexes in the lower extremities and a nondermatomal sensory loss.

Neuroimaging is shown in Figs. 15-4-1–15-4-2.

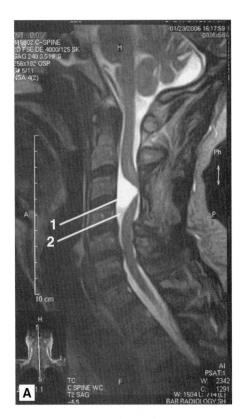
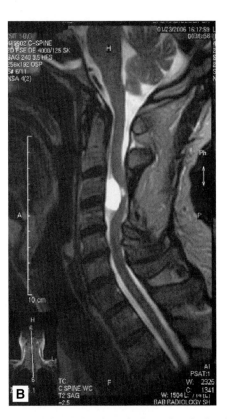

FIG. 15-4-1   A and **B.** T2 sagittal MRI demonstrating large arachnoid cyst (1) involving the spinal canal at the level of C3-4. The cyst contains higher T2 signal than the surrounding CSF (2) The majority of the mass is anterior, displacing the cord posterior and laterally.

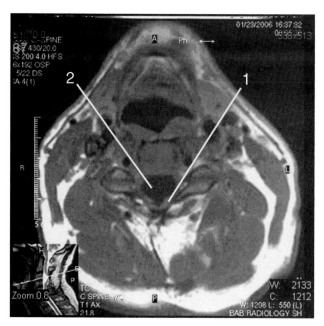

FIG. 15-4-2 The severe cord compression (1) caused by the cyst (2) is apparent when viewed in this axial T1 image.

Clinical-Radiological Diagnosis: Arachnoid cyst.

KEY FACTS

The pathogenesis of arachnoid cysts is unknown. Intradural arachnoid cysts are most commonly posterior to spinal cord and located in the thoracic region.

REFERENCE

Kazan S, Ozdemir O, Akyuz M, Tuncer R. Spinal intradural arachnoid cysts located anterior to the cervical spinal cord. Report of two cases and review of the literature. *J Neurosurg.* 1999 Oct;91(2 Suppl):211–5.

CASE 15-5

A 63-year-old man is evaluated for progressive loss of strength in the lower extremities over the past 3 years associated with recent onset of loss of sphincter control. Neurological examination shows spastic paraparesis associated with hypoesthesia of the lower extremities. Paresis and hypoesthesia, as well as increased tendon reflexes, are asymmetric, being more severe on the left side. A Babinski sign is present on the left. A lumbar tap does not show evidence of multiple sclerosis or other inflammatory, degenerative or neoplastic disorders. A spine MRI is obtained.

Neuroimaging is shown in Figs. 15-5-1–15-5-2.

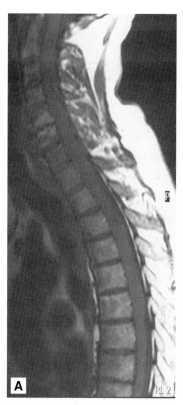

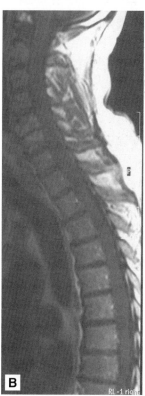

FIG. 15-5-1 Spine T1 MRI does not show a focal lesion. **A.** On a sagittal cut without contrast, the spinal cord is diffusely swollen, especially in the thoracic segment. **B.** No areas of enhancement can be appreciated, following the injection of intravenous contrast (gadolinium).

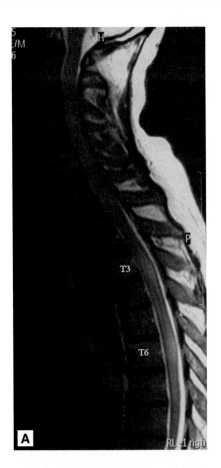

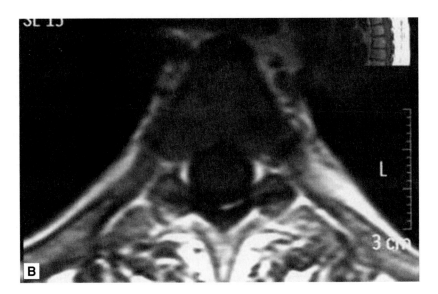

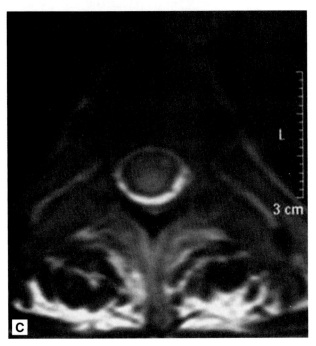

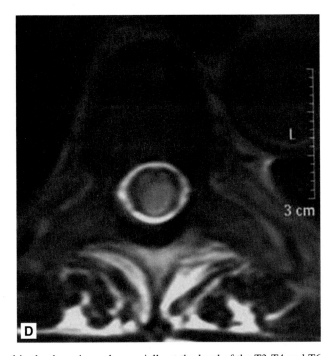

FIG. 15-5-2 A. Sagittal T2 MRI shows a diffuse hyperintense signal in the thoracic cord, especially at the level of the T3-T4 and T6 vertebral bodies **B.** Axial T1 postcontrast cuts show again lack of gross signal abnormalities and contrast enhancement **C.** High signal changes within the spinal cord are easily appreciated on T2 imaging at the level of the upper edge of T4 and the body of T6 **D.** The axial cut also shows a rounded lesion displaying a homogeneous hyperintense signal. This lesion occupies the central and posterior two-thirds of the spinal cord and is slightly eccentric to the left. Spots of high T2 signal can be seen also in the anterior and lateral part of the spinal cord outside the rounded lesion. The MRI remains completely unchanged after a course of IV steroids.

Clinical-Radiological Diagnosis: Diffuse spinal cord glioma.

KEY FACTS

This clinical history could be associated with a wide range of intra- and extra-axial spinal lesions. Among the intraxial spinal cord lesions, gliomas, multiple sclerosis, and lymphoma are most commonly associated with this clinical picture. The history of a slowly progressive neurological deficit, the presence of diffuse signal changes within the spinal cord on T2 imaging without evidence of contrast enhancement on T1 imaging, and the absence of findings on a lumbar tap as well as the lack of changes on the MR following steroid administration are strongly suggestive of a spinal cord diffuse low grade glioma. This diagnosis was confirmed by a surgical specimen (WHO Grade II diffuse glioma).

CASE 15-6

A 41-year-old man was diagnosed with a thoracolumbar myxopapillary ependymoma many years ago. He recently presented to his neurosurgeon with increasing difficulty walking, and mild lower extremity weakness on examination.

Neuroimaging is shown in Figs. 15-6-1–15-6-4.

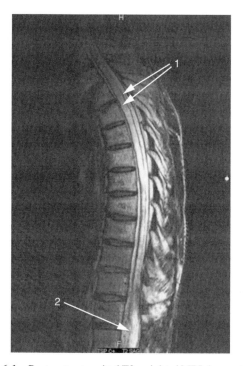

FIG. 5-6-1 Postcontrast sagittal T2 weighted MRI demonstrating an intramedullary spinal cord cyst throughout the entire length of the spinal cord. Spinal cord tissue is visible anterior and posterior to the cyst (1). The ependymoma is labeled by arrow (2).

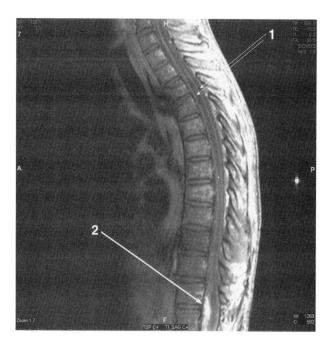

FIG. 15-6-2 The ependymoma is shown to be clearly enhancing in this post-contrast T1 MRI. A syrinx with surrounding spinal cord (1) is apparent.

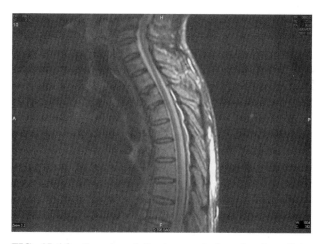

FIG. 15-6-3 Two days following surgical exploration of the ependymoma and removal of arachnoid adhesions the cyst has nearly entirely resolved.

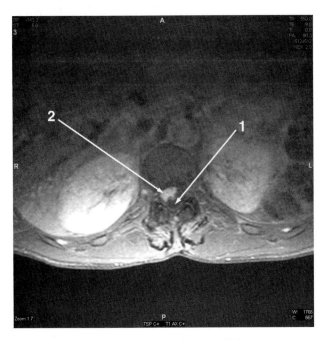

FIG. 15-6-4 The enhancing ependymoma (2) is apparent anteriorly and laterally to the lower spinal cord (1).

Clinical-Radiological Diagnosis: Syrinx secondary to thoracolumbar myxopapillary ependymoma.

KEY FACTS

Any lesion which obstructs CSF flow may cause a syrinx. MRI is the best imaging modality for radiologically studying the progress of a syrinx.

REFERENCE

Tanghe H.L.J. Magnetic resonance imaging in syringomyelia. *Acta Neurochir.* 1995;134:93–9.

Chapter 16

MULTIPLE SCLEROSIS AND AUTOIMMUNE DISORDERS

CASE 16-1

A 32-year-old woman presents with a 3-day history of worsening leg weakness and urinary incontinence.

Exam is significant for a mild-to-moderate spastic paraparesis and impaired joint proprioception in the toes.

Neuroimaging is shown in Figs. 16-1-1–16-1-2.

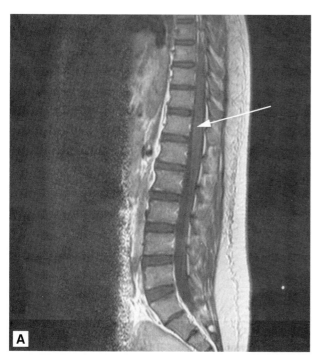
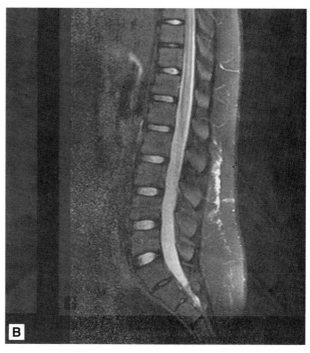

FIG. 16-1-1 **A.** Sagittal T2 **B.** T2 with fat suppression (STIR) **C.** T1 postcontrast images. The findings show abnormal high T2/low T1 signal (white arrow) within the spinal cord. The lesion is nonenhancing. These findings suggest a demyelinating process. *(Continued)*

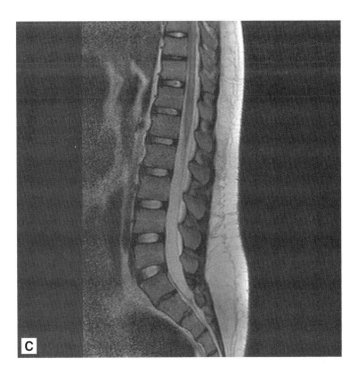

FIG. 16-1-1   *(Continued)*

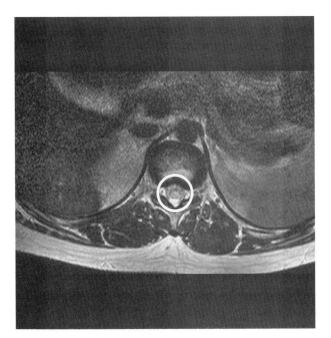

FIG. 16-1-2   An axial T2 image shows that the abnormal signal is present throughout most of the white matter.

Clinical-Radiologic Diagnosis: Transverse myelitis.

KEY FACTS

Transverse myelitis is often associated with multiple sclerosis, but the differential diagnosis includes many etiologies including other autoimmune disorders, Devic's disease, vasculitis, infections, and tumor.

REFERENCE

Scotti G, Gerevini S. Diagnosis and differential diagnosis of acute transverse myelopathy. The role of neuroradiological investigations and review of the literature. *Neurol Sci.* 2001;22(2): S69–73.

Chapter 17

TRAUMA

CASE 17-1

A 32-year-old man dove into a shallow swimming pool. He immediately felt pain in his neck and a loss of sensation in his lower extremities. Both of his lower extremities were also weak, worse on the left than the right.

Neuroimaging is shown in Figs. 17-1-1–17-1-4.

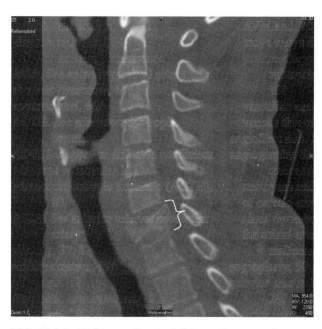

FIG. 17-1-1 Reformatted sagittal CT scan demonstrating comminuted, compressed fracture of the C7 vertebral body.

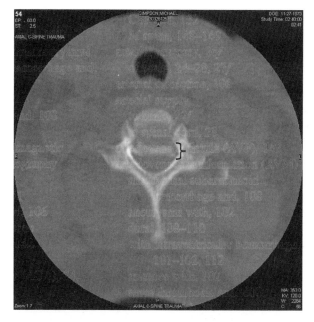

FIG. 17-1-2 Retropulsion of the posterior fragment has narrowed the spinal canal.

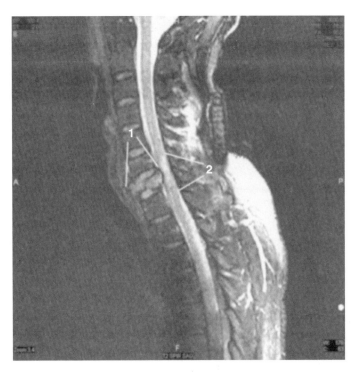

FIG. 17-1-3   Sagittal MRI showing the fracture (1), compressing the spinal cord (2) which displays abnormal high T2 signal.

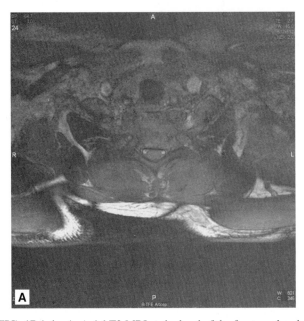
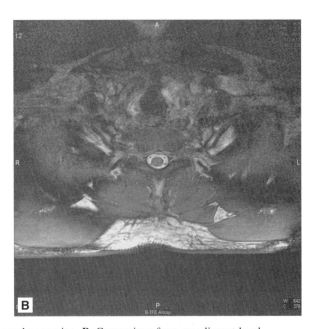

FIG. 17-1-4   **A.** Axial T2 MRI at the level of the fracture showing canal narrowing. **B.** Comparison from an adjacent level.

Clinical-Radiological Diagnosis: C7 traumatic fracture.

KEY FACTS

Bony structures are more easily visualized with CT, while MRI is superior for directly imaging the spinal cord.

CASE 17-2

A 45-year-old roofer had used marijuana shortly before going to work. Under the influence of the drug he lost his footing and fell approximately 25 feet to the ground. In the emergency room he mentioned severe neck pain, but denied weakness or sensory symptoms.

Neuroimaging is shown in Figs. 17-2-1–17-2-2.

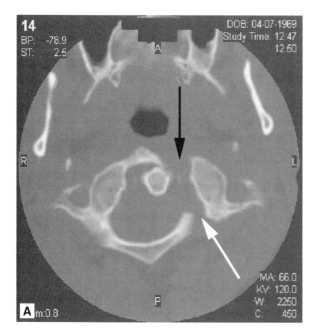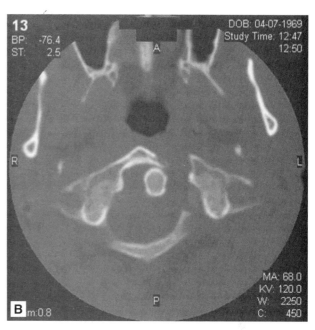

FIG. 17-2-1 **A** and **B.** Axial CT scan demonstrating a C1 fracture involving the left anterior (black arrow) and posterior (white arrow) arch. There is approximately 7–8 mm lateral distraction of the fracture fragments at the anterior arch.

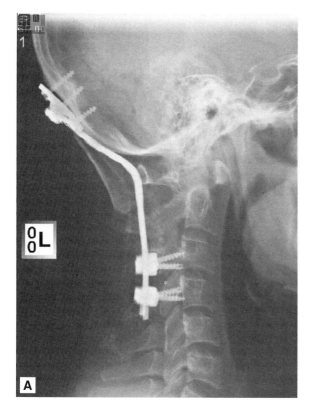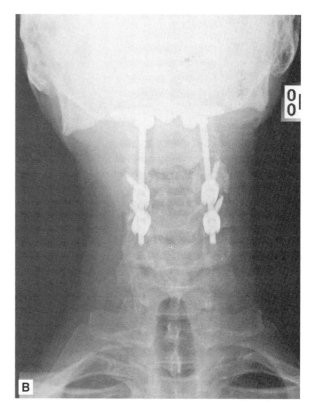

FIG. 17-2-2 **A** and **B.** X-rays following posterior fixation with screws, plates, and rods.

Clinical-Radiological Diagnosis: Traumatic cervical spine fracture.

KEY FACTS

CT scanning is preferable to plain films for imaging the spine of trauma patients. This is particularly important in cases of high cervical trauma.

REFERENCE

Bagley LJ. Imaging of spinal trauma. *Radiol Clin North Am.* 2006;44(1):1–12, vii.

Chapter 18

SPINE INFECTIONS

CASE 18-1

A 63-year-old man with a history of cholecystitis, low back pain, fevers, and bilateral lower extremity weakness.

Neuroimaging is shown in Figs. 18-1-1 to 18-1-4.

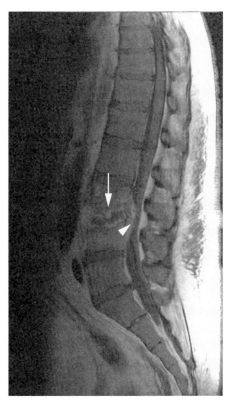

FIG. 18-1-1 Postcontrast fat saturated T1 weighted image of the lumbar spine shows enhancement in the L3/4 intervertebral disk space (white arrow), with an enhancing lesion that extends posteriorly into the epidural space (white arrowhead).

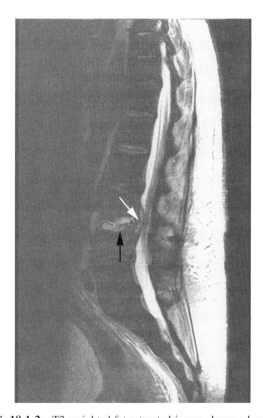

FIG. 18-1-2 T2 weighted fat saturated image shows edema in the L3 and L4 vertebral bodies as well as high signal in the L3-4 intervertebral disk space (black arrow). There is a hyperintense epidural mass as well (white arrow).

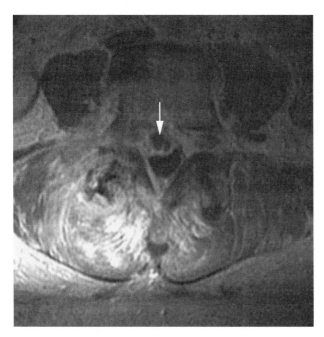

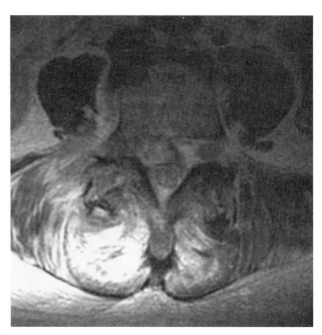

FIG. 18-1-3 Axial post gadolinium image from a different patient shows a ring enhancing mass lesion in the epidural space (white arrow). The differential diagnosis for this finding in isolation includes an epidural abscess or a herniated disk fragment.

FIG. 18-1-4 Axial T2 weighted image (from the same patient in Fig. 18-1-3) shows a high signal well circumscribed epidural lesion in a right paracentral location.

Clinical-Radiological Diagnosis: Epidural Abscess from discitis/osteomyelitis.

KEY FACTS

An epidural abscess can result from adjacent discitis/osteomyelits, hematogenous seeding, or direct infection such as recent instrumentation, an adjoining psoas abscess, or a decubitus ulcer. Characteristically discitis is characterized by high signal within the disk space on MRI, with enhancement after gadolinium, and adjacent bone marrow edema. Epidural abscess may be characterized by enhancing soft tissue phlegmon, or a true organized abscess with a necrotic center.

Plain films and CT may show signs of end plate erosion, and loss of normal disk height.

REFERENCE

Reihaus E, Waldbaur H, Seeling W. Spinal epidural abscesses: a meta-analysis of 915 patients. *Neurosurg Rev.* 2000;232:175–204.

Chapter 19

GENETIC AND DEGENERATIVE DISORDERS

CASE 19-1

An otherwise healthy 14-year-old girl was noticed to have an abnormal curvature of the spine during

routine clinical examination. Surgical correction was performed.

Neuroimaging is shown in Figs. 19-1-1–19-1-3.

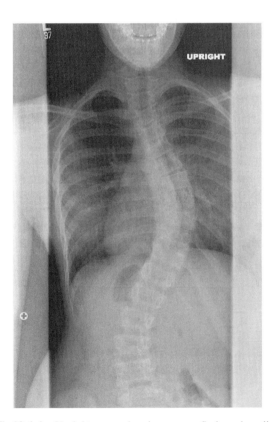

FIG. 19-1-1 Upright x-ray showing severe S-shaped scoliosis with dextrocurvature at the mid-thoracic spine and levocurvature at the mid-lumbar spine.

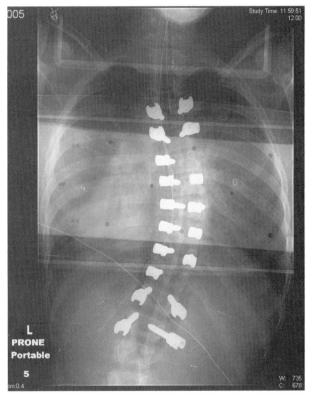

FIG. 19-1-2 Intraoperative film following placement of pedicle screws at multiple levels from the mid-thoracic to the upper lumbar.

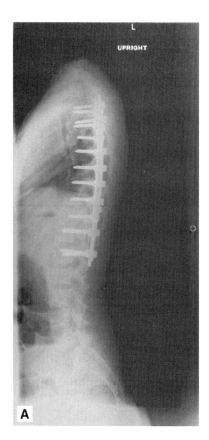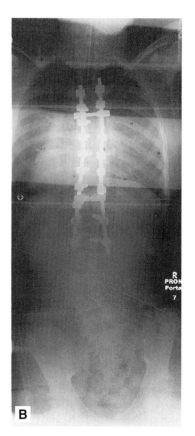

FIG. 19-1-3 A. Lateral **B.** Posterior-anterior views showing the scoliosis correction with rods in place.

Clinical-Radiological Diagnosis: Idiopathic Scoliosis.

KEY FACTS

Plain radiographs remain the standard for initial diagnosis and monitoring of scoliosis. MRI or CT may be useful for evaluating the underlying cause of the deformity and treatment planning.

REFERENCE

Thomsen M, Abel R. Imaging in scoliosis from the orthopaedic surgeon's point of view. *Eur J Radiol.* 2006;58(1):41–7.

CASE 19-2

The patient is a 10-year-old girl with bladder and bowel paralysis, hyperreflexia, spasticity, and sensory deficits of the lower extremities.

Neuroimaging is shown in Figs. 19-2-1–19-2-3.

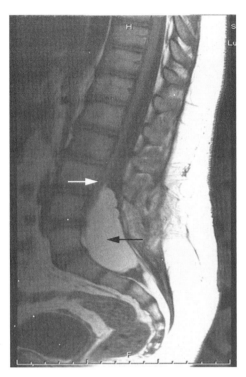

FIG. 19-2-1 A sagittal T1 weighted image shows a fat containing mass lesion (black arrow) with an associated low lying conus medullaris (white arrow), located at L4. There is expansion of the lumbosacral spinal canal from this fat containing lesion.

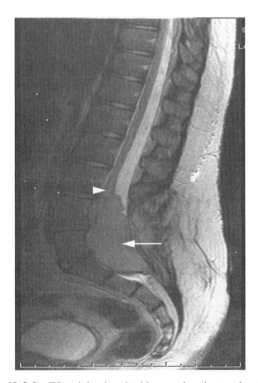

FIG. 19-2-2 T2 weighted sagittal image also shows a low lying conus medullaris at the L4 level (white arrowhead). A fat containing mass is again seen (white arrow), which is low signal intensity because of the application of a fat saturation pulse.

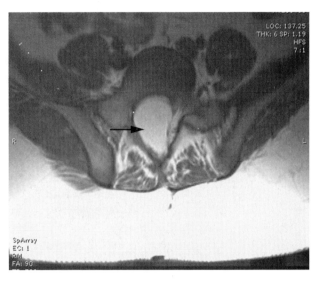

FIG. 19-2-3 Axial T1 weighted image shows a defect in the posterior elements, with a fat containing mass (black arrow) and nerve roots extruding from the defect.

Clinical-Radiological Diagnosis: Lipomyelomeningocele with sacral spina bifida.

KEY FACTS

A lumbosacral lipomyelomeningocele is herniation of an intradural and intramedullary fat containing mass through a bony defect. When detected in infants, these lesions are usually associated with a large subcutaneous mass. Associated cutaneous stigmata can include skin dimples and hemangiomas. Management consists of early surgical intervention to prevent loss of neurological function, even in patients who are asymptomatic at the time of presentation.

REFERENCES

Kanev PM, Bierbrauer KS. Reflections on the natural history of lipomyelomeningocele. *Pediatr Neurosurg.* 1995;22:137–140.
Kanev PM, Lemire RJ, Loeser JD, Berger MS. Management and long term follow up review of children with lipomyelomeningocele, 1952–1987. *J Neurosurg.* 1990;73:48–52.

Chapter 20

DEGENERATIVE SPINE DISEASE

CASE 20-1

The patient is a 70-year-old man with right leg sciatica in a posterolateral distribution radiating into the dorsum of his right foot.

Neuroimaging is shown in Figs. 20-1-1–20-1-2.

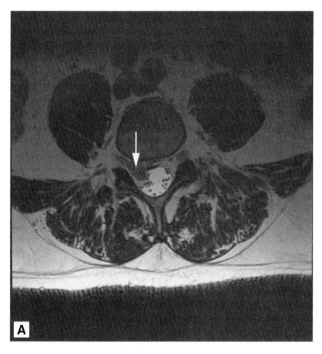
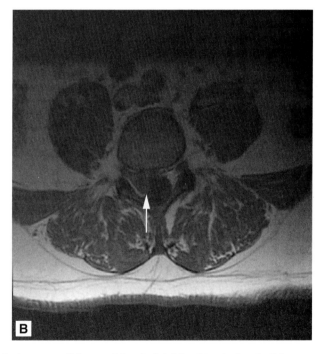

FIG. 20-1-1   A. Axial T1 **B.** T2; weighted images show a large mass isointense to disk material at the L4-5 level impinging the L5 nerve root on the right (white arrow).

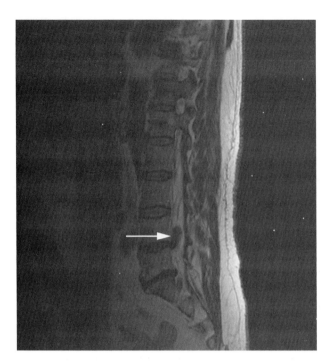

FIG. 20-1-2 Sagittal T2 weighted image shows a large pro-truded disk fragment originating from the L4-5 intervertebral disk space (white arrow). Note that the end plates of the superior and inferior vertebral bodies are normal in appearance.

Clinical-Radiologic Diagnosis: Disk herniation with a protruded disk fragment.

KEY FACTS

Intervertebral disk herniations are a common cause of radicular pain. A disk herniation is by definition a focal displacement of disk material (less than 50% of disk cir-cumference). In the lumbar spine, herniated disks most commonly occur in the lower levels (L4-5 and L5-S1). A herniated fragment with a broad based attachment to the intervertebral disk is a protrusion. A herniated disk with a narrow base or no attachment is an extruded disk frag-ment. A herniated disk with no contact with the parent intervertebral disk is a sequestered disk fragment.

CASE 20-2

A 76-year-old man reports progressive loss of strength in his legs associated with stiffness and difficulties in walking.

He also has neck pain radiating to the shoulders and arms bilaterally. There is no history of trauma. Neurological examination reveals spastic paraparesis with increased deep tendon reflexes and presence of pathological reflexes (Babinski and Hoffman) and clonus. Bilateral 4/5 weakness in the triceps and absence of tricipital reflex at the elbow. Plain films of the cervical spine (AP view plus lateral view in flexion and extension) are unremark-able. A cervical spine MRI is obtained.

Neuroimaging is shown in Figs. 20-2-1 to 20-2-2.

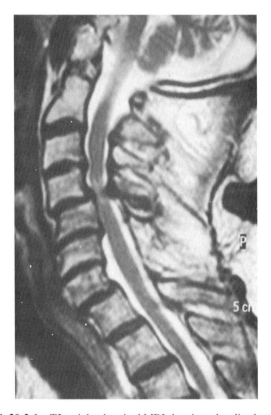

FIG. 20-2-1 T2 weighted sagittal MRI showing a localized steno-sis with anterior and posterior compression on the spinal cord at the level C4-C5. The anterior compression is mostly related to mis-alignment of the vertebral bodies, with C4 shifting anteriorly on C5. The posterior compression is related to hypertrophy of the ligamen-tum flavum, appreciated from C2 to C5. This hypertrophy is partic-ularly severe at the C4 level, where no white CSF signal can be appreciated and the dark signal of the flavum touches the spinal cord. The spinal cord at the junction C4-C5 is markedly compressed and displays a hyperintense signal suggesting localized damage.

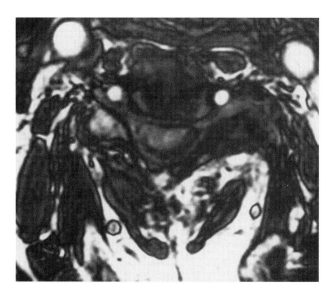

FIG. 20-2-2 T2 weighted axial cut taken at C4-C5 level. A hyperintense signal can be appreciated inside the spinal cord. No CSF signal can be appreciated, while posteriorly the dark signal of the hypertrophic ligamentum flavum surrounds the spinal cord. Anteriorly a moderate degree of hypertrophy of the posterior longitudinal ligament can be appreciated.

Clinical-Radiological Diagnosis: Cervical stenosis with myelopathy.

KEY FACTS

Cervical stenosis is a common cause of myelopathy in the elderly. Frequent findings are diffuse hypertrophy of the ligamentum flavum and/or instability of the vertebral bodies. This case shows that even a localized hypertrophy of the flavum (in this case at C4-C5 level) can cause spinal cord damage and severe neurological disability.

CASE 20-3

A 35-year-old woman undergoes a surgical procedure including instrumentation and fusion for low back pain. Immediately after the operation she notices pain shooting down her right lower extremity.

Neuroimaging is shown in Fig. 20-3-1.

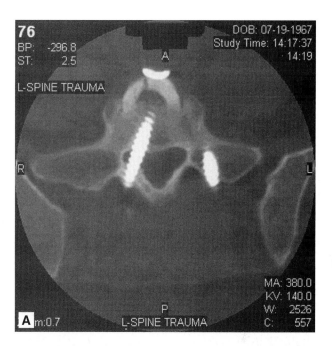

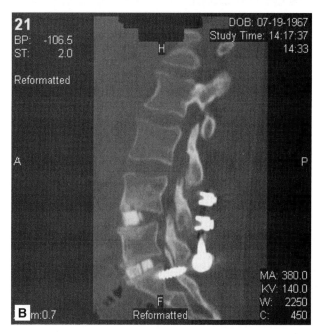

FIG. 20-3-1 A, B, and **C.** These images are from a CT scan performed several months after the procedure. The clinically most relevant finding is the medial breach of the right S1 pedicle screw. The screw has clearly entered the canal in the position where the nerve root would normally lie. *(Continued)*

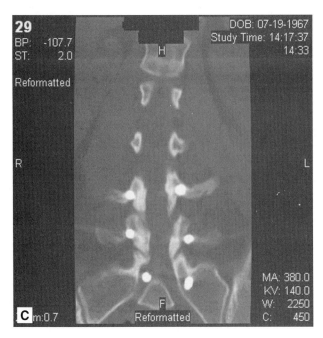

FIG. 20-3-1 *(Continued)*

Clinical-Radiological Diagnosis: S1 radiculopathy secondary to pedicle screw breach.

KEY FACTS

Spine stabilization with pedicle screws and rods has become very common over the past several years. The screws must be placed "blindly" for the most part; although intraoperative x-rays can provide AP and lateral views and the surgeon can probe the hole with an instrument. CT guidance and neurophysiological testing appear to be useful to prevent this unfortunate outcome.

Chapter 21

BENIGN MRI AND CT FINDINGS

CASE 21-1

A 35-year-old woman with no other medical problems has persistent back pain associated with bilateral sciatic pain. The pain intensity is rated as modest and is not associated with neurological abnormalities. However the patient has an anxious personality and believes that "something is wrong." Her family physician decides to obtain a lumbar spine MRI without contrast to reassure the patient.

Neuroimaging is shown in Fig. 21-2-1.

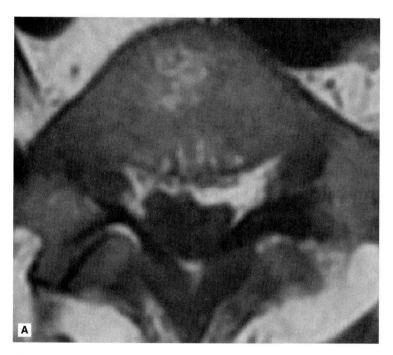
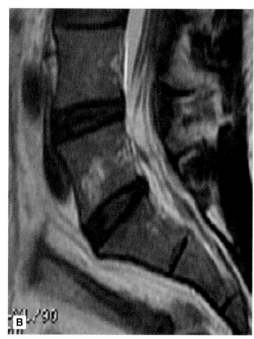

FIG. 21-2-1 A. Non contrast axial and **B.** Sagittal T2 weighted MRI show the presence of a hyperintense region in the antero-inferior part of the L5 vertebral body. Similar findings were also present on axial and sagittal T1 weighted images. A modest protrusion of the L5-S1 disk is apparent.

Clinical-Radiological Diagnosis: Vertebral body hemangioma.

KEY FACTS

Benign vertebral body hemangiomas are a common incidental finding in patients undergoing spinal MRI. This lesion is not a cause of spinal instability, is not evolutive, and does not require any treatment or further study. The original complaint of back pain with a sciatic component is likely to be unrelated to the hemangioma.

INDEX

Page numbers followed by *f* or *t* indicate figures or tables, respectively.